Paramedic Care
Principles & Practice
Special Patients

Workbook

Fourth Edition

ROBERT S. PORTER

REVISED BY

TONY CRYSTAL, SC.D., EMT-P

EMS Program Coordinator
Richland Community College
Decatur, Illinois

BRYAN E. BLEDSOE, DO, FACEP, FAAEM, EMT-P

Professor of Emergency Medicine
Director, Prehospital and Disaster Medicine Fellowship
University of Nevada School of Medicine
Attending Emergency Physician
University Medical Center of Southern Nevada
Medical Director, MedicWest Ambulance
Las Vegas, Nevada

ROBERT S. PORTER, MA, EMT-P

Senior Advanced Life Support Educator
Madison County Emergency Medical Services
Canastota, New York

RICHARD A. CHERRY, MS, NREMT-P

Director of Training
Northern Onondaga Volunteer Ambulance
Liverpool, New York

D0074157

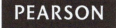

PEARSON

Boston   Columbus   Indianapolis   New York   San Francisco   Upper Saddle River
Amsterdam   Cape Town   Dubai   London   Madrid   Milan   Munich   Paris   Montréal   Toronto
Delhi   Mexico City   São Paulo   Sydney   Hong Kong   Seoul   Singapore   Taipei   Tokyo

Publisher: *Julie Levin Alexander*
Publisher's Assistant: *Regina Bruno*
Editor-in-Chief: *Marlene McHugh Pratt*
Senior Managing Editor for Development: *Lois Berlowitz*
Editorial Project Manager: *Triple SSS Press Media
    Development, Inc.*
Assistant Editor: *Jonathan Cheung*
Director of Marketing: *David Gesell*
Marketing Manager: *Brian Hoehl*
Marketing Specialist: *Michael Sirinides*
Managing Editor for Production: *Patrick Walsh*
Production Liaison: *Faye Gemmellaro*
Production Editor: *Muralidharan Krishnamurthy/S4Carlisle
    Publishing Services*
Manufacturing Manager: *Ilene Sanford*
Cover Design: *Kathryn Foot*
Cover Image: © *corepics/Shutterstock*
Composition: *S4Carlisle Publishing Services*
Cover and Interior Printer/Binder: *Edwards Brothers Malloy*

NOTICE ON CPR AND ECC

The national standards for cardiopulmonary resuscitation (CPR) and emergency cardiovascular care (ECC) are reviewed and revised on a regular basis and may change slightly after this manual is printed. It is important that you know the most current procedures for CPR and ECC, both for the classroom and your patients. The most current information may be obtained from the appropriate credentialing agency.

NOTICE ON CARE PROCEDURES

It is the intent of the authors and publisher that this Workbook be used as part of a formal Paramedic program taught by qualified instructors and supervised by a licensed physician. The procedures described in this Workbook are based upon consultation with EMS and medical authorities. The authors and publisher have taken care to make certain that these procedures reflect currently accepted clinical practice; however, they cannot be considered absolute recommendations.

The material in this Workbook contains the most current information available at the time of publication. However, federal, state, and local guidelines concerning clinical practices, including, without limitation, those governing infection control and universal precautions, change rapidly. The reader should note, therefore, that the new regulations may require changes in some procedures.

It is the responsibility of the reader to familiarize himself or herself with the policies and procedures set by federal, state, and local agencies as well as the institution or agency where the reader is employed. The authors and the publisher of this Workbook disclaim any liability, loss, or risk resulting directly or indirectly from the suggested procedures and theory, from any undetected errors, or from the reader's misunderstanding of the text. It is the reader's responsibility to stay informed of any new changes or recommendations made by any federal, state, and local agency as well as by his or her employing institution or agency.

Brady
is an imprint of

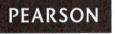

www.bradybooks.com

10 9 8 7 6 5 4 3 2 1

ISBN 10: 0-13-211146-2
ISBN 13: 978-0-13-211146-1

Dedication

This workbook is dedicated to the important people in your life: your wife/husband, mother, father, sister, brother . . . and friends who support you and the time and passion you devote to Emergency Medical Service.
Without them, this endeavor would be lonely and much less rewarding.

–ROBERT S. PORTER

CONTENTS

INTRODUCTION

Welcome to the self-instructional Workbook for *Paramedic Care: Principles & Practice*. This Workbook is designed to help guide you through an educational program for initial or refresher training that follows the guidelines of the 2009 *National EMS Education Standards*. The Workbook is designed to be used either in conjunction with your instructor or as a self-study guide you use on your own.

This Workbook features many different ways to help you learn the material necessary to become a paramedic, as described next.

Features

Review of Chapter Objectives

Each chapter of *Paramedic Care: Principles & Practice* begins with objectives that identify the important information and principles addressed in the chapter reading. To help you identify and learn this material, each Workbook chapter reviews the important content elements addressed by these objectives as presented in the text.

Case Study Review

Each chapter of *Paramedic Care: Principles & Practice* includes a case study, introducing and highlighting important principles presented in the chapter. The Workbook reviews these case studies and points out much of the essential information and many of the applied principles they describe.

Content Self-Evaluation

Each chapter of *Paramedic Care: Principles & Practice* presents an extensive narrative explanation of the principles of paramedic practice. The Workbook chapter (or chapter section) contains between 10 and 50 multiple-choice questions to test your reading comprehension of the textbook material and to give you experience taking typical emergency medical service examinations.

Special Projects

The Workbook contains several projects that are special learning experiences designed to help you remember the information and principles necessary to perform as a paramedic. Special projects include contacting local agencies and services, Internet research, and a variety of other exercises.

Content Review

The Workbook provides a comprehensive review of the material presented in Volume 6 of *Paramedic Care: Principles & Practice*. After the last text chapter has been covered, the Workbook presents an extensive content self-evaluation component that helps you recall and build upon the knowledge you have gained by reading the text, attending class, and completing the earlier Workbook chapters.

Patient Scenario Flash Cards

At the end of this Workbook are scenario flash cards, which are designed to help you practice the processes of investigating both the chief complaint and the past medical history. Each card contains the dispatch information and results of the scene size-up and then prompts you to inquire into either the patient's major symptoms or past medical history.

How to Use This Self-Instructional Workbook

The self-instructional Workbook accompanying *Paramedic Care: Principles & Practice* may be used as directed by your instructor or independently by you during your course of instruction. The following recommendations are intended to guide you in using the Workbook independently.

- Examine your course schedule and identify the appropriate text chapter or other assigned reading.

- Read the assigned chapter in *Paramedic Care: Principles & Practice* carefully. Do this in a relaxed environment, free of distractions, and give yourself adequate time to read and digest the material. The information presented in *Paramedic Care: Principles & Practice* is often technically complex and demanding, but it is very important that you comprehend it. Be sure that you read the chapter carefully enough to understand and remember what you have read.

- Carefully read the Review of Chapter Objectives at the beginning of each Workbook chapter (or section). This material includes both the objectives listed in *Paramedic Care: Principles & Practice* and narrative descriptions of their content. If you do not understand or remember what is discussed from your reading, refer to the referenced pages and reread them carefully. If you still do not feel comfortable with your understanding of any objective, consider asking your instructor about it.

- Reread the case study in *Paramedic Care: Principles & Practice*, and then read the Case Study Review in the Workbook. Note the important points regarding assessment and care that the Case Study Review highlights and be sure that you understand and agree with the analysis of the call. If you have any questions or concerns, ask your instructor to clarify the information.

- Take the Content Self-Evaluation at the end of each Workbook chapter (or section), answering each question carefully. Do this in a quiet environment, free from distractions, and allow yourself adequate time to complete the exercise. Correct your self-evaluation by consulting the answers at the back of the Workbook, and determine the percentage you have answered correctly (the number you got right divided by the total number of questions). If you have answered most of the questions correctly (85 to 90 percent), review those that you missed by rereading the material on the pages listed in the answer key and be sure you understand which answer is correct and why. If you have more than a few questions wrong (less than 85 percent correct), look for incorrect answers that are grouped together. This suggests that you did not understand a particular topic in the reading. Reread the text dealing with that topic carefully, and then retest yourself on the questions you got wrong. If incorrect answers are spread throughout the chapter content, reread the chapter and retake the Content Self-Evaluation to ensure that you understand the material. If you don't understand why your answer to a question is incorrect after reviewing the text, consult with your instructor.

- In a similar fashion, complete the exercises in the Special Projects section of the Workbook chapters (or sections). These exercises are specifically designed to help you learn and remember the essential principles and information presented in *Paramedic Care: Principles & Practice*.

- When you have completed this volume of *Paramedic Care: Principles & Practice* and its accompanying Workbook, prepare for a course test by reviewing both the text in its entirety and your class notes. Then take the Content Review examination in the Workbook. Again, review your score and any questions you have answered incorrectly by referring to the text and rereading the page or pages where the material is presented. If you note groupings of wrong answers, review the entire range of pages or the full chapter they represent.

If, during your completion of the Workbook exercises, you have any questions that either the textbook or Workbook doesn't answer, write them down and ask your instructor about them. Prehospital emergency medicine is a complex and complicated subject, and answers are not always black and white. It is also common for different EMS systems to use differing methods of care. The questions you bring up in class, and your instructor's answers to them, will help you expand and complete your knowledge of prehospital emergency medical care.

GUIDELINES TO BETTER TEST-TAKING

The knowledge you will gain from reading the textbook, completing the exercises in the Workbook, listening in your paramedic class, and participating in your clinical and field experience will prepare you to care for patients who are seriously ill or injured. However, before you can practice these skills, you will have to pass several classroom written exams and your state's certification exam. Your performance on these exams will depend not only on your knowledge but also on your ability to answer test questions correctly. The following guidelines are designed to help your performance on tests and to better demonstrate your knowledge of pre-hospital emergency care.

1. Relax and be calm during the test.

A test is designed to measure what you have learned and to tell you and your instructor how well you are doing. An exam is not designed to intimidate or punish you. Consider it a challenge, and just try to do your best. Get plenty of sleep before the examination. Avoid coffee or other stimulants for a few hours before the exam, and be prepared.

Reread the text chapters, review the objectives in the Workbook, and review your class notes. It might be helpful to work with one or two other students and ask each other questions. This type of practice helps everyone better understand the knowledge presented in your course of study.

2. Read the questions carefully.

Read each word of the question and all the answers slowly. Words such as "except" or "not" may change the entire meaning of the question. If you miss such words, you may answer the question incorrectly even though you know the right answer.

Example:
The art and science of emergency medical services involves all of the following EXCEPT

    A. sincerity and compassion.
    B. respect for human dignity.
    C. placing patient care before personal safety.
    D. delivery of sophisticated emergency medical care.
    E. none of the above.

The correct answer is C, unless you miss the "EXCEPT."

3. Read each answer carefully.

Read each and every answer carefully. Although the first answer may be absolutely correct, so may the rest, and thus the best answer might be "all of the above."

Example:
Indirect medical direction is considered to be

    A. treatment protocols.
    B. training and education.
    C. quality assurance.
    D. chart review.
    E. all of the above.

Although answers A, B, C, and D are each correct, the best and only acceptable answer is "all of the above," E.

4. Delay answering questions you don't understand and look for clues.

When a question seems confusing or you don't know the answer, note it on your answer sheet and come back to it later. This will ensure that you have time to complete the test. You will also find that other questions in the test may give you hints to answer the one you've skipped over. It will also prevent you from being frustrated with an early question and letting it affect your performance.

Example:

Upon successful completion of a course of training as an EMT-P, most states will

    A.   certify you. (correct)

    B.   license you.

    C.   register you.

    D.   recognize you as a paramedic.

    E.   issue you a permit.

Another question, later in the exam, may suggest the right answer:

The action of one state in recognizing the certification of another is called

    A.   reciprocity. (correct)

    B.   national registration.

    C.   licensure.

    D.   registration.

    E.   extended practice.

5. Answer all questions.

Even if you do not know the right answer, do not leave a question blank. A blank question is always wrong, whereas a guess might be correct. If you can eliminate some of the answers as wrong, do so. It will increase the chances of a correct guess.

A multiple-choice question with five answers gives a 20 percent chance of a correct guess. If you can eliminate one or more incorrect answers, you increase your odds of a correct guess to 25 percent, 33 percent, and so on. An unanswered question has a 0 percent chance of being correct.

Just before turning in your answer sheet, check to be sure that you have not left any items blank.

Example:

When a paramedic is called by the patient (through the dispatcher) to the scene of a medical emergency, the medical direction physician has established a physician/patient relationship.

    A.   True

    B.   False

A true/false question gives you a 50 percent chance of a correct guess.

The hospital health professional(s) responsible for sorting patients as they arrive at the emergency department is/are usually the

    A.   emergency physician.

    B.   ward clerk.

    C.   emergency nurse.

    D.   trauma surgeon.

    E.   both A and C. (correct)

Chapter 1

Gynecology

Review of Chapter Objectives

In each chapter of the workbook, we identify the objectives and the important elements of the text content. You should review these items and refer to the pages listed if any points are not clear.

After reading this chapter, you should be able to:

1. Define key terms introduced in this chapter. p. 2

Knowing and being able to apply the key terms in each chapter is critical to understanding chapter concepts. Write the list of key terms. Then write the definition of each one in your own words. Check your understanding by confirming the definitions in the text glossary. Correct any misunderstandings. Create a study aid by writing each key term on the front of an index card and the definition on the back. Use the cards to quiz yourself, or to have someone quiz you.

2. Relate the anatomy and physiology of the female reproductive system to the assessment and management of patients with gynecologic disorders. pp. 3–8

A thorough understanding of the anatomy and physiology of the female reproductive system will allow you to better understand, recognize, and treat gynecologic emergencies when they arise. The most important female reproductive organs are internal and are located within the pelvic cavity. These include the ovaries, fallopian tubes, uterus, and vagina, which are essential to reproduction. The external genitalia have accessory functions, in that they protect body openings and play an important role in sexual functioning. These include the perineum, mons pubis, labia, clitoris, and urethra.

A monthly hormonal cycle prepares the uterus to receive a fertilized egg. The first two weeks of the cycle (known as the proliferative phase) are dominated by estrogen, causing the uterine lining to thicken. In response to a surge of luteinizing hormone, ovulation takes place and an egg is released from the ovary. The secretory phase is the stage of the menstrual cycle immediately surrounding ovulation. If the egg is not fertilized, the woman's estrogen level drops sharply while the progesterone level dominates. Uterine vascularity increases in anticipation of implantation. If fertilization does not occur, estrogen and progesterone levels fall, triggering vascular changes and leaving the endometrium ischemic. The ischemic endometrium is shed during the menstrual phase (menstruation), along with a discharge of blood, mucus, and cellular debris. Menstrual flow usually lasts three to five days, with an average blood loss of 50 mL.

3. Use a process of clinical reasoning to guide and interpret the patient assessment and management process for patients with specific gynecologic complaints. pp. 8–10

The most common gynecological complaints are abdominal pain and vaginal bleeding. Complete your initial assessment in the usual manner and then proceed with a focused history and physical exam. Specific questions will need to be asked that are pertinent to reproductive function and dysfunction. If pertinent, be sure to gather information about the patient's obstetrical history, including pregnancies and deliveries. It is important to document the date of the patient's last menstrual period (LMP). You should also ask what form of birth control, if any, she uses and, if pertinent, whether she uses it regularly. Pay particular attention to the physical exam, which will be limited to assessment of the abdomen and potentially (in the presence of serious bleeding) inspection of the patient's perineum. Gently auscultate and palpate the abdomen. Be sure to note the color, character, and volume of any blood lost. An internal vaginal exam should never be performed in the prehospital setting.

4. **Adapt the scene size-up, primary assessment, patient history, secondary assessment, and use of monitoring technology to meet the needs of patients with complaints and presentations related to gynecologic disorders.**   p. 10

As with any emergency situation, vital signs are useful clues as to your patient's status as well as the severity of the condition. Be alert for early signs of shock or a positive tilt test, both of which point to significant blood loss. If possible, estimate blood loss. The use of two sanitary pads per hour is considered significant bleeding.

Management of gynecological emergencies is focused on supportive care. Rely on your initial assessment guidance in your decision making about oxygen therapy, ventilatory support, and vascular access. In the presence of shock, follow your local protocols for fluid resuscitation and use of the pneumatic anti-shock garment (PASG). In cases of heavy bleeding, do not pack dressings in the vagina. Continue to monitor the patient's status and bleeding en route to definitive care. Equally important is the psychological support that you give your patient. Protect her modesty and privacy.

5. **Adapt the scene size-up, primary assessment, patient history, secondary assessment, and use of monitoring technology to meet the needs of patients with complaints and presentations related to sexual assault.**   pp. 13–14

The victim of sexual assault is a unique patient with unique needs. Your patient needs emergency medical treatment and psychological support. Your patient also needs to have legal evidence gathered. Your objectivity is essential, as your attitude may affect long-term psychological recovery. As a rule, victims of sexual abuse should not be questioned about the incident in the field. Do not ask questions about specific details of the assault. It is not important, from the standpoint of prehospital care, to determine whether penetration took place. Do not inquire about the patient's sexual practices. Confine your questions to the physical injuries the patient received. Even well-intentioned questions may lead to guilt feelings in the patient.

6. **Demonstrate concern for the psychosocial needs of patients with gynecologic emergencies and sexual assault.**   pp. 10–14

The psychological response of sexual assault victims is widely variable. The victim of sexual assault may be withdrawn or hysterical. Some use denial, anger, or fear as defense mechanisms. Approach the patient calmly and professionally. Allay the patient's fear and anxiety. Respond to the patient's feelings but be aware of your own. If the patient is incompletely dressed, a cover should be offered. Respect the patient's modesty. Explain all procedures and obtain the patient's permission before beginning them. Avoid touching the patient other than to take vital signs or examine other physical injuries. Do not examine the genitalia unless there is life-threatening hemorrhage.

7. **Relate the pathophysiology of specific gynecologic disorders, including pelvic inflammatory disease, ovarian cysts, cystitis, mittelschmerz, endometritis, endometriosis, ectopic pregnancy, nontraumatic vaginal bleeding, and genital trauma, to the priorities of patient assessment and management.**

Pelvic Inflammatory Disease   pp. 10–11

Pelvic inflammatory disease (PID), the most common cause of nontraumatic abdominal pain in women in the childbearing years, is an infection of the female reproductive tract that is most commonly caused by gonorrhea or chlamydia. Predisposing factors include multiple sexual partners, prior history of PID, recent gynecological procedure, or an intrauterine device (IUD). The patient will look acutely ill and will often present with diffuse lower abdominal pain, and may also have fever, chills, nausea, vomiting, and possibly a foul-smelling vaginal discharge. The patient may also walk with a shuffling gait due to pain. Blood pressure may be normal, and fever may or may not be present. Palpation of the lower abdomen usually elicits moderate to severe pain. The primary management in the field is supportive care and a position of comfort during transport. If the patient appears septic, administer oxygen and initiate intravenous (IV) therapy.

Ovarian Cysts   p. 11

Cysts are fluid-filled pockets, and, when they develop in the ovary, they can rupture and be a source of abdominal pain. The rupture spills a small amount of blood into the abdomen, irritating the peritoneum and causing abdominal pain and rebound tenderness. Usually the patient complains of moderate to severe unilateral abdominal pain that may radiate to the back; it may be associated with vaginal bleeding. The patient may also report pain during intercourse or a delayed menstrual period. The primary management in the field is supportive care and a position of comfort during transport.

Cystitis   p. 11

A bacterial infection of the urinary bladder (cystitis) is a common cause of abdominal pain that may be accompanied by urinary frequency, dysuria, and a low-grade fever. The pain is generally located just above the symphysis pubis unless the infection has spread to the kidneys, in which case there is likely to be flank pain as well. The primary management in the field is supportive care and a position of comfort during transport.

Mittelschmerz   pp. 11–12

Midcycle abdominal pain may accompany ovulation. Unilateral lower-quadrant pain is usually self-limited and may be accompanied by midcycle spotting. Treatment is symptomatic.

Endometritis   p. 12

Endometritis, an infection of the uterine lining, is an occasional complication of miscarriage, childbirth, or gynecological procedures. Commonly reported signs and symptoms include mild to severe lower abdominal pain, a bloody and foul-smelling discharge, and fever that may mimic the signs of PID. The primary management in the field is supportive care and a position of comfort during transport. If the patient appears septic, administer oxygen and initiate IV therapy.

Endometriosis   p. 12

Endometriosis is a condition in which endometrial tissue is found outside the uterus. Most commonly, it is found in the abdomen and pelvis. Regardless of the site, the tissue responds to the hormones of the menstrual cycle, thus bleeding in a cyclic manner. The condition is most common in women between ages 30 and 40 and is rare in postmenopausal women. The patient complains of dull, cramping pelvic pain, usually related to menstruation. The primary management in the field is supportive care and a position of comfort during transport.

Ectopic Pregnancy   p. 12

Ectopic pregnancy is the implantation of a fetus outside of the uterus, most commonly in the fallopian tubes. Patients usually report severe unilateral abdominal pain that may radiate to the shoulder on the affected side, a late or missed menstrual period, and sometimes vaginal bleeding. As the fetus develops, the tube can rupture, triggering a massive, life-threatening hemorrhage. Absorb the bleeding but do not pack the vagina. Ectopic pregnancy is a surgical emergency, and the primary management in the field is supportive care and a position of comfort during transport, as well as oxygen administration and IV therapy for fluid resuscitation.

Nontraumatic Vaginal Bleeding   p. 12

Nontraumatic vaginal hemorrhage is rarely encountered in the prehospital setting unless it is severe. Do not presume that such bleeding is due to normal menstrual flow. Most commonly, it is due to a spontaneous abortion (miscarriage) and is associated with cramping abdominal pain and the passage of clots and tissue. Other possible causes include cancerous lesions, PID, or the onset of labor. Absorb bleeding but do not pack the vagina. The primary management in the field is supportive care and a position of comfort for the patient, as well as oxygen administration and IV therapy for fluid resuscitation. If the bleeding is due to miscarriage, this will likely be a significant emotional event for your patient, so your kind and considerate care is important.

Genital Trauma   pp. 13–14

Traumatic vaginal bleeding may result from sexual assault, blunt-force injuries to the lower abdomen, seat-belt injuries, objects inserted into the vagina, self-attempts at abortion, and lacerations following childbirth. Bleeding in such cases should be managed by direct pressure over a laceration or a cold pack applied to a hematoma. Never pack the vagina. Provide expedited transport to the hospital, with oxygen administration and IV access as necessary.

8. **Observe special considerations for evidence preservation when dealing with a patient who has been sexually assaulted.**   pp. 13–14

Preservation of physical evidence is important. When the patient arrives at the hospital, a physician or sexual assault nurse examiner will complete a sexual assault examination to gather physical evidence. Consider the patient a crime scene and protect that scene. Handle clothing as little as possible, if at all. If you must remove clothing, bag separately each item that must be bagged. Do not cut through any tears or holes in the clothing. Place bloody articles in brown paper bags. Do not examine the perineal area. If the assault took place within the hour or the patient is bleeding, put an absorbent pad under the patient's hips to collect that evidence. If you cover the patient with a sheet or blanket, turn that over to the hospital as evidence. Do not allow patients to change their clothes, bathe, or douche before the medical examination. Do not allow patients to comb their hair, brush their teeth, or clean their fingernails. Do not clean wounds, if at all possible. If you must initiate care on scene, avoid disruption of the crime scene.

9. **Observe special considerations in documentation of calls involving sexual assault.**   p. 14

When completing your patient care report, state the patient's remarks accurately. Objectively state your observations of the patient's physical condition, environment, or torn clothing. Document any evidence turned over to the hospital staff and the name of the individual to whom you gave it. Do not include your opinions as to whether rape occurred.

Case Study Review

Reread the case study on pages 2 and 3 in Paramedic Care: Special Patients; *then, read the following discussion.*

This case study draws attention to the assessment and management of a sexual assault patient in the prehospital setting. Sexual assault continues to represent the most rapidly growing violent crime in the United States, so it is likely that you will encounter these patients in the course of your career.

In this scenario, the paramedics meet their patient in the care of the park police officer who found her. Stephanie has been allowed to cover herself and afforded privacy before the arrival of the medics. Being mindful of the psychological aspects of her care, the medic explains every necessary procedure and asks her permission before any action is initiated. Recognizing the need to preserve potential evidence, the medic keeps the blanket around Stephanie. The initial and rapid trauma assessments revealed no significant injuries or immediate life threats. The paramedic consistently gave control to Stephanie and reassured her that she was safe now. She was transported to the hospital for evaluation by the sexual assault nurse examiner.

©2013 Pearson Education, Inc.
Paramedic Care: Principles & Practice, Vol. 6, 4th Ed.

Content Self-Evaluation

MULTIPLE CHOICE

_____ 1. Thickening of the endometrium in preparation for implantation of a fertilized egg is stimulated by
  A. follicle-stimulating hormone and luteinizing hormone.
  B. luteinizing hormone and estrogen.
  C. estrogen and progesterone.
  D. progesterone and follicle-stimulating hormone.
  E. estrogen and follicle-stimulating hormone.

_____ 2. Ovulation occurs at approximately day 14 of the menstrual cycle in response to a surge of
  A. follicle-stimulating hormone.   D. progesterone.
  B. luteinizing hormone.   E. all of the above.
  C. estrogen.

_____ 3. All of the following are phases of the menstrual cycle EXCEPT the
  A. ischemic phase.   D. excretory phase.
  B. proliferative phase.   E. menstrual phase.
  C. secretory phase.

_____ 4. The average blood loss associated with menstruation is
  A. 5 mL.   D. 150 mL.
  B. 50 mL.   E. 250 mL.
  C. 100 mL.

_____ 5. The variety of physical signs and symptoms associated with the changing hormonal levels of the menstrual cycle is known as
  A. menarche.   D. premenstrual syndrome.
  B. menstruation.   E. hormonal surge.
  C. menopause.

_____ 6. The term used to describe the number of times a woman has been pregnant is *parity*.
  A. True
  B. False

_____ 7. A palpable abdominal mass found midway between the symphysis pubis and the umbilicus in the lower abdomen of a 25-year-old woman is most likely to be a(n)
  A. tumor.
  B. intrauterine pregnancy of 5 months' gestation.
  C. intrauterine pregnancy of 4 months' gestation.
  D. intrauterine pregnancy of 3 months' gestation.
  E. ovarian cyst.

_____ 8. Pelvic inflammatory disease is most often caused by
  A. gonorrhea and chlamydia.   D. chlamydia and streptococcus.
  B. streptococcus and staphylococcus.   E. HIV and staphylococcus.
  C. gonorrhea and HIV.

_____ 9. Midcycle abdominal pain associated with ovulation is known as
  A. endometriosis.   D. cystitis.
  B. PID.   E. mittelschmerz.
  C. a miscarriage.

_____ 10. Endometriosis is an infection of the uterine lining.
  A. True
  B. False

_____ 11. The most effective means to control vaginal hemorrhage is to apply direct pressure to the perineum.
A. True
B. False

_____ 12. All of the following signs and symptoms are associated with endometritis EXCEPT
A. history of gynecological procedure.
B. severe abdominal pain.
C. bloody, foul-smelling discharge.
D. bradycardia.
E. fever.

_____ 13. All of the following signs and symptoms are associated with a ruptured ovarian cyst EXCEPT
A. dyspareunia.
B. severe abdominal pain.
C. fever.
D. delayed menstrual period.
E. irregular bleeding.

_____ 14. If a female patient presents with severe unilateral abdominal pain that radiates to the shoulder on one side, a missed menstrual period, and vaginal bleeding, you should suspect
A. mittelschmerz.
B. ectopic pregnancy.
C. PID.
D. endometriosis.
E. cystitis.

_____ 15. The prehospital priorities for care of the sexual assault victim include all of the following EXCEPT
A. examining for perineal tears.
B. determining if life-threatening injuries exist.
C. providing emotional support.
D. preserving evidence.
E. protecting the patient's privacy.

Label the Diagram

In the spaces provided, write the names of the organs of the female reproductive system marked A through E on the following diagram.

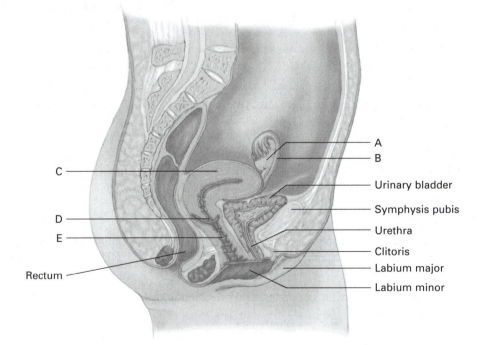

©2013 Pearson Education, Inc.
Paramedic Care: Principles & Practice, Vol. 6, 4th Ed.

A. _____

B. _____

C. _____

D. _____

E. _____

Special Project

Problem Solving: Abdominal Pain

You are dispatched for "woman with abdominal pain." Your patient is a 26-year-old female who looks acutely ill and complains of severe abdominal pain.

1. Given this information, what would you attempt to determine when gathering a focused history?

_____ _____

_____ _____

_____ _____

_____ _____

Having obtained the history, you perform a physical exam. Your findings include the following:

- tachypnea
- tachycardia
- pale, cool, diaphoretic skin
- narrowed pulse pressure
- vaginal bleeding or discharge
- abdominal exam: masses, distention, guarding, localized tenderness, rebound

2. Based on this information, provide a differential diagnosis for this patient.

_____ _____

_____ _____

_____ _____

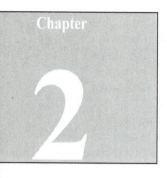

2

Obstetrics

Review of Chapter Objectives

In each chapter of the workbook, we identify the objectives and the important elements of the text content. You should review these items and refer to the pages listed if any points are not clear.

After reading this chapter, you should be able to:

1. Define key terms introduced in this chapter.   **p. 18**

Knowing and being able to apply the key terms in each chapter is critical to understanding chapter concepts. Write the list of key terms. Then write the definition of each one in your own words. Check your understanding by confirming the definitions in the text glossary. Correct any misunderstandings. Create a study aid by writing each key term on the front of an index card and the definition on the back. Use the cards to quiz yourself, or to have someone quiz you.

2. Relate the anatomy and physiology of pregnancy and fetal development to the assessment and management of patients with obstetric presentations.   **pp. 19–24**

The first two weeks of the menstrual cycle are dominated by the hormone estrogen, which causes the endometrium (the inner lining of the uterus) to thicken and become engorged with blood. In response to a surge of luteinizing hormone (LH) and follicle-stimulating hormone (FSH), ovulation, or release of an egg (ovum) from the ovary, takes place. If the egg has been fertilized, it becomes implanted in the uterus and pregnancy begins. If the egg has not been fertilized, menstruation (discharge of blood, mucus, and cellular debris from the endometrium) takes place 14 days after ovulation. If fertilization occurs, the ovum begins cellular division immediately, which continues as it moves through the fallopian tube to the uterus. The ovum then becomes a blastocyst. The blastocyst normally implants in the thickened uterine lining, which has been prepared for implantation by the hormone progesterone, where the fetus and placenta subsequently develop.

Approximately three weeks after fertilization, the placenta develops on the uterine wall at the site where the blastocyst attached. The placenta, known as the "organ of pregnancy," is a temporary, blood-rich structure that serves as the lifeline for the developing fetus. It transfers heat while exchanging oxygen and carbon dioxide, delivering nutrients and carrying away wastes. When expelled from the uterus following the birth of the child, the placenta and accompanying membranes are called the afterbirth. The placenta is connected to the fetus by the umbilical cord that normally contains two arteries and one vein. The umbilical vein transports oxygenated blood to the fetus, and the umbilical arteries return relatively deoxygenated blood to the placenta.

The fetus develops within the amniotic sac, sometimes called the "bag of waters" (BOW). This thin-walled membranous covering holds the amniotic fluid that surrounds and protects the fetus during intrauterine development. The presence of amniotic fluid allows for fetal movement within the uterus and serves to cushion and protect the fetus from trauma. Although it may rupture earlier, the amniotic sac usually breaks during labor, and the amniotic fluid or "water" flows out of the vagina. This is called rupture of the membranes (ROM).

The physiologic changes associated with pregnancy are due to an altered hormonal state, the mechanical effects of the enlarging uterus and its significant vascularity, and the increasing metabolic demands on the maternal system. The most significant pregnancy-related changes occur in the uterus. Other changes occurring in the reproductive system include the formation of a mucous plug in the cervix that protects the developing fetus and helps to prevent infection. The breasts enlarge and become more nodular as the mammary glands increase in number and size in preparation for lactation.

During pregnancy, maternal oxygen demands increase. To meet this need, progesterone causes a decrease in airway resistance. This results in a 20 percent increase in oxygen consumption and a 40 percent increase in tidal volume. There is only a slight increase in respiratory rate. Cardiac output increases throughout pregnancy, peaking at 6 to 7 liters/minute by the time the fetus is fully developed. The maternal blood volume increases by 45 percent and, although both red blood cells and plasma increase, there is slightly more plasma, resulting in a relative anemia. Because of the increase in blood volume, the pregnant female may suffer an acute blood loss of 30 to 35 percent without a significant change in vital signs. The maternal heart rate increases by 10 to 15 beats/minute. Blood pressure decreases slightly during the first two trimesters of pregnancy and then rises to near nonpregnant levels during the third trimester.

Nausea and vomiting are common in the first trimester as a result of hormone levels and changed carbohydrate needs. Peristalsis is slowed, so delayed gastric emptying is likely and bloating or constipation is common. As the uterus enlarges, abdominal organs are compressed, and the resulting compartmentalization of abdominal organs makes assessment difficult.

Renal blood flow increases during pregnancy. The glomerular filtration rate increases by nearly 50 percent in the second trimester and remains elevated throughout the remainder of the pregnancy. The urinary bladder gets displaced anteriorly and superiorly, increasing the potential for rupture. Urinary frequency is common, particularly in the first and third trimesters,

Loosened pelvic joints caused by hormonal influences account for the waddling gait that is often associated with pregnancy. As the uterus enlarges and the mother's center of gravity changes, postural changes take place to compensate for anterior growth, causing low back pain.

3. **Use a process of clinical reasoning to guide and interpret the patient assessment and management process for patients with specific obstetric presentations.**   p. 24

The initial approach to the obstetric patient should be the same as for the nonobstetric patient, with special attention paid to the developing fetus. Complete the primary assessment quickly, and then obtain essential obstetric information. The SAMPLE history will allow you to gain specific information about the mother's situation as well as her pertinent medical history.

You will want to obtain information about the pregnancy, such as the mother's gravidity and parity, the length of gestation, and the estimated due date, if known. In addition, you should determine whether the patient has had any cesarean sections or any gynecologic or obstetric complications in the past. It is also important to ascertain whether the patient has had any prenatal care. A general overview of the patient's current state of health is important. Pay particular attention to current medications and drug and/or medication allergies.

4. **Adapt the scene size-up, primary assessment, patient history, secondary assessment, and use of monitoring technology to meet the needs of patients with complaints and presentations related to obstetric conditions.**

Diabetes   pp. 24–25

Previously diagnosed diabetes can become unstable during pregnancy due to altered insulin requirements. Diabetics are at increased risk of developing preeclampsia and hypertension (discussed later in this chapter). Pregnancy may also accelerate the progression of vascular disease complications of diabetes. It is not uncommon for pregnant diabetics to have problems with fluctuating blood sugar levels, causing hypoglycemic or hyperglycemic episodes. In addition, many patients develop diabetes during pregnancy (gestational diabetes). Pregnant diabetics cannot be managed with oral hypoglycemic agents because these drugs tend to cross the placenta and affect the fetus. Therefore, all pregnant diabetics are placed on insulin,

©2013 Pearson Education, Inc.
Paramedic Care: Principles & Practice, Vol. 6, 4th Ed.

if their blood sugar levels cannot be controlled by diet alone. It has been shown that maintaining careful control of the mother's blood sugar between 70 and 120 mg/dL reduces risks to the mother and fetus.

Diabetes also affects the infant. Infants of diabetic mothers, especially those with poorly controlled blood sugar levels, tend to be large. This complicates delivery. Such infants also may have trouble maintaining body temperature after birth and may be subject to hypoglycemia. Babies born to diabetic mothers are also at increased risk of congenital anomalies (birth defects).

Heart Disease p. 25

During pregnancy, cardiac output increases up to 30 percent. Patients who have serious preexisting heart disease may develop congestive heart failure in pregnancy. When confronted by a pregnant patient in obvious or suspected heart failure, inquire about preexisting heart disease or murmurs. It is important to be aware, however, that most patients develop a quiet systolic flow murmur during pregnancy. This is caused by increased cardiac output and is rarely a source of concern.

Hypertension p. 25

Hypertension is also aggravated by pregnancy. Generally, blood pressure is lower in pregnancy than in the nonpregnant state. However, women who were borderline hypertensive before becoming pregnant may become dangerously hypertensive when pregnant. Furthermore, many common blood pressure medications cannot be used during pregnancy. In addition, preeclampsia may contribute to maternal hypertension. Persistent hypertension may adversely affect the placenta, thus compromising the fetus as well as placing the mother at increased risk for stroke, seizure, or renal failure.

Seizure Disorders p. 25

Most women with a history of seizure disorders controlled by medication have uneventful pregnancies and deliver healthy babies. However, women who have poorly controlled seizure disorders are likely to have increased seizure activity during pregnancy. Medications to control seizures are commonly administered throughout the pregnancy.

Neuromuscular Disorders p. 25

Disabilities associated with neuromuscular disorders, such as multiple sclerosis, may be aggravated by pregnancy. However, it is more common that pregnant women enjoy remission of symptoms during pregnancy and a slight increase in relapse rate during the postpartum period. The strength of uterine contractions is not diminished in these patients. Also, their subjective sensation of pain is often less than that seen in other patients.

Pain p. 25

If the patient is in pain, try to determine when the pain started and whether its onset was sudden or slow. Also, attempt to define the character of the pain—its duration, location, and radiation, if any. It is especially important to determine whether the pain is occurring on a regular basis.

Vaginal Bleeding p. 25

The presence of vaginal bleeding or spotting is a major concern in an obstetric patient. Ask about events immediately prior to the start of bleeding. You also need to gain information about the color, amount, and duration of bleeding. To assess the amount of bleeding, count the number of sanitary pads or tampons used. If your patient is passing clots or tissue, save this material for evaluation. In addition, question the patient about the presence of other vaginal discharge, as well as the color, amount, and duration.

Active Labor p. 25

When confronted with a patient in active labor, assess whether the mother feels the need to push or has the urge to move her bowels. Determine whether the patient thinks her membranes have ruptured.

When examining a pregnant patient, first estimate the date of the pregnancy by measuring the fundal height. The fundal height is the distance from the pubic symphysis to the top of the uterine fundus. Each centimeter of fundal height roughly corresponds to a week of gestation. If the fundus is just palpable above the pubic symphysis, the pregnancy is about 12 to 16 weeks' gestation. When the uterine fundus reaches the umbilicus, the pregnancy is about 20 weeks. As pregnancy reaches term, the fundus is palpable near the xiphoid process. If fetal movement is felt when the abdomen is palpated, the pregnancy is at least 20 weeks. Fetal heart tones can be heard by stethoscope at approximately 18 to 20 weeks. The normal fetal heart rate ranges from 140 to 160 beats per minute.

Occasionally, it may be helpful to perform orthostatic vital signs. First, obtain the blood pressure and pulse rate after the patient has rested for 5 minutes in the left lateral recumbent position. Then repeat the vital signs with the patient sitting up or standing. A drop in the blood pressure level of 15 mmHg or more, or an increase in the pulse rate of 20 beats per minute or more, is considered significant and should be reported and documented.

You may need to examine the genitals to evaluate any vaginal discharge, the progression of labor, or the presence of a prolapsed cord, an umbilical cord that comes out of the uterus ahead of the fetus. If, during the physical examination, the patient reports that she feels the need to push, or if she feels as though she must move her bowels, examine her for crowning. Crowning is an indication of impending delivery. Examine for crowning only during a contraction. Do not perform an internal vaginal examination in the field.

5. **Demonstrate concern for the psychosocial needs of patients with obstetric conditions.** p. 26

The first consideration for managing emergencies in obstetric patients is to remember that you are, in fact, caring for two patients, the mother and the fetus. Fetal well-being is dependent on maternal well-being. Also keep in mind that your calm, professional demeanor and caring attitude will go a long way in reducing the emotional stress during any obstetric emergency. Remember to protect your patient's privacy and maintain her modesty.

6. **Identify indications of imminent obstetric delivery.** p. 35

It is generally preferable to transport the mother unless delivery is imminent. Several factors must be taken into consideration when making this decision. They include the patient's number of previous pregnancies, the length of labor during the previous pregnancies, the frequency of contractions, the maternal urge to push, and the presence of crowning. Some women have rapid labor and may be completely dilated in a short period of time. The maternal urge to push or the presence of crowning indicates that delivery is imminent. In such cases, the infant should be delivered at the scene or in the ambulance.

7. **Perform the steps of caring for the mother and newborn in complicated and uncomplicated newborn delivery.** p. 26

The physiologic priorities for obstetric emergencies are identical to those for any other emergency situation. Focus your efforts on maintaining the airway, breathing, and circulation. Administer oxygen, if needed, to correct hypoxia. Initiate intravenous access by using a large-bore catheter in a large vein and consider fluid resuscitation based on your local protocols. If your patient is bleeding or showing signs of shock, establish two IV lines. Cardiac monitoring is also appropriate. Place your patient in a position of comfort, but remember that the left lateral recumbent position is preferred after the 24th week.

If pain is the primary complaint, administer analgesics such as morphine. However, analgesics should be used with caution as they can alter your ability to assess a deteriorating condition as well as other changes in patient status and may negatively affect the fetus. Nitrous oxide is the preferred analgesic in pregnancy, but narcotics are acceptable.

When transport is indicated, transport immediately to a hospital that is capable of managing emergency obstetric and neonatal care. Report the situation to the receiving hospital prior to your arrival, as emergency department personnel may want to summon obstetrics department staff to assist with patient care.

8. **Recognize abnormal deliveries that cannot be managed in the prehospital setting.** p. 35

Certain factors should prompt immediate transport, despite the threat of delivery. These include prolonged rupture of membranes (>24 hours), as prolonged time between rupture and delivery often leads to fetal infection; abnormal presentation, such as breech or transverse; prolapsed cord; or fetal distress,

©2013 Pearson Education, Inc.
Paramedic Care: Principles & Practice, Vol. 6, 4th Ed.

as evidenced by fetal bradycardia or meconium staining (the presence of meconium, the first fetal stools, in the amniotic fluid). The presence of multiple fetuses may also contribute to your decision to transport.

9. Relate the pathophysiology of specific obstetric disorders, including trauma in pregnancy, abortion, ectopic pregnancy, preterm labor, placenta previa, abruptio placenta, hypertensive disorders of pregnancy, abnormal fetal presentations in labor, and postpartum complications, to the priorities of patient assessment and management.

Trauma
pp. 26–27

Pregnant victims of major trauma are more susceptible to life-threatening injury than are nonpregnant victims because of the increased vascularity of the gravid uterus. Trauma is the most frequent, nonobstetric cause of death in pregnant women. Paramedics should anticipate the development of shock based on the mechanism of injury rather than waiting for overt signs and symptoms. Because of the cardiovascular changes of pregnancy, overt signs of shock are late and inconsistent. Fetal death may result from death of the mother, separation of the placenta from the uterine wall, maternal shock, uterine rupture, or fetal head injury.

Trauma management essentials include the following: apply a C-collar to provide cervical stabilization and immobilize on a long backboard; administer oxygen if the patient is hypoxic; initiate two large-bore IVs for crystalloid administration per protocol; transport tilted to the left to minimize supine hypotension; reassess frequently; and monitor the fetus.

Abortion
p. 27

Abortion, the expulsion of the fetus prior to 20 weeks' gestation, is the most common cause of bleeding in the first and second trimesters of pregnancy. The terms abortion and miscarriage can be used interchangeably. Generally, abortion is considered as termination of pregnancy at maternal request, and miscarriage is considered as an accident of nature. Medically, the term abortion applies to both kinds of fetal loss. About half of all abortions are due to the result of fetal chromosomal anomalies. Other causes include maternal reproductive system abnormalities, maternal use of drugs, placental defects, or maternal infections.

The patient experiencing an abortion is likely to report cramping abdominal pain and a backache. She is also likely to report vaginal bleeding, which is often accompanied by the passage of clots and tissue.

Place the patient who is experiencing an abortion in a position of comfort. Treat for shock with oxygen therapy (if hypoxic) and IV access for fluid resuscitation. As mentioned earlier, any tissue or large clots should be retained and given to emergency department personnel. An abortion is generally a very sad occurrence. Provide emotional support to the parents.

Ectopic Pregnancy
pp. 27–28

The term *ectopic pregnancy* refers to the abnormal implantation of the fertilized egg outside the uterus. Predisposing factors in the development of ectopic pregnancy include scarring of the fallopian tubes due to pelvic inflammatory disease (PID), a previous ectopic pregnancy, or previous pelvic or tubal surgery, such as a tubal ligation. Other factors include endometriosis or use of an intrauterine device (IUD) for birth control.

Ectopic pregnancy most often presents as abdominal pain, which starts out as diffuse tenderness and then localizes as a sharp pain in the lower abdominal quadrant on the affected side. As the intra-abdominal bleeding continues, the abdomen becomes rigid and the pain intensifies and is often referred to the shoulder on the affected side. The pain is often accompanied by syncope, vaginal bleeding, and shock. Assume that any female woman of childbearing age with lower abdominal pain is experiencing an ectopic pregnancy.

Ectopic pregnancy poses a significant life threat to the mother. Transport this patient immediately, as surgery is often required to resolve the situation. Interim care measures should include oxygen therapy (if the patient is hypoxic) and IV access for fluid resuscitation.

Placenta Previa

pp. 28–29

Placenta previa occurs as a result of abnormal implantation of the placenta on the lower half of the uterine wall, resulting in partial or complete coverage of the cervical opening. Although the exact cause of placenta previa is unknown, certain predisposing factors are commonly seen. These factors include a previous history of placenta previa, multiparity, or increased maternal age. Other factors include the presence of uterine scars from cesarean sections, a large placenta, or defective development of blood vessels in the uterine wall.

The patient with placenta previa is usually a multigravida in her third trimester of pregnancy. She may have a history of prior placenta previa or of bleeding early in the current pregnancy. The onset of painless bright red vaginal bleeding, which may occur as spotting or recurrent hemorrhage, is the hallmark of placenta previa.

Because of the potential for profuse hemorrhage, you should treat for shock. Administer oxygen if the patient is hypoxic and initiate intravenous access. Additionally, continue to monitor the maternal vital signs and fetal heart tones. Because the definitive treatment is delivery of the fetus by cesarean section, it is imperative to transport the patient to a hospital with obstetric surgical capability.

Abruptio Placenta

pp. 29–30

Abruptio placentae, or the premature separation (abruption) of a normally implanted placenta from the uterine wall, poses a potential life threat for both mother and fetus. Although the cause of abruptio placentae is unknown, predisposing factors include multiparity, maternal hypertension, trauma, cocaine use, increasing maternal age, and history of abruption in previous pregnancy.

The presenting signs and symptoms of abruptio placentae vary depending on the extent and character of the abruption. Partial abruptions can be marginal or central. Marginal abruption is characterized by vaginal bleeding but no increase in pain. In central abruption, the placenta separates centrally and the bleeding is trapped between the placenta and the uterine wall, or "concealed," so there is no vaginal bleeding. However, there is a sudden sharp, tearing pain and development of a stiff, boardlike abdomen. In complete abruptio placentae there is massive vaginal bleeding and profound maternal hypotension.

Abruptio placentae is a life-threatening obstetrical emergency. Immediate intervention to maintain maternal oxygenation and perfusion is imperative. Immediately place two large large-bore intravenous lines and begin fluid resuscitation. Position your patient in the left lateral recumbent position. Transport immediately to a hospital with available surgical obstetric and high-risk neonatal care.

Preeclampsia

pp. 30–31

Preeclampsia is the most common hypertensive disorder seen in pregnancy. Preeclampsia is a progressive disorder that is usually categorized as mild or severe. Seizures (or coma) develop in its most severe form, known as eclampsia. Preeclampsia is defined as an increase in systolic blood pressure by 30 mmHg and/or a diastolic increase of 15 mmHg over baseline on at least two occasions at least 6 hours apart. Mild preeclampsia is characterized by hypertension, edema, and protein in the urine. Severe preeclampsia progresses rapidly, with maternal blood pressures reaching 160/110 or higher, while the edema becomes generalized and the amount of protein in the urine increases significantly. Other commonly seen signs and symptoms in the severe state include headache, visual disturbances, hyperactive reflexes, and the development of pulmonary edema, along with a dramatic decrease in urine output.

The patient who is hypertensive and shows other signs and symptoms of preeclampsia, such as edema, headaches, and visual disturbances, should be treated quickly. Keep the patient calm and dim the lights. Place the patient in the left lateral recumbent position and quickly carry out the primary assessment. Begin an IV of normal saline. Transport the patient rapidly, without lights or sirens. If the blood pressure is dangerously high (diastolic > 110), medical direction may request the administration of hydralazine (Apresoline) or similar antihypertensives that are safe for use in pregnancy. If the transport time is long, the administration of magnesium sulfate may also be ordered.

Eclampsia

pp. 30–31

Eclampsia, the most serious manifestation of the hypertensive disorders of pregnancy, is characterized by generalized tonic-clonic (major motor) seizure activity. Eclampsia is often preceded by visual disturbances, such as flashing lights or spots before the eyes.

If the patient has already suffered a seizure or a seizure appears to be imminent, keep the patient calm and dim the lights. Place the patient in the left lateral recumbent position and quickly carry out the primary assessment. Begin an IV of normal saline, administer oxygen (if the patient is hypoxic), and manage the airway appropriately. Administer a bolus dose of magnesium sulfate (2 to 5 g diluted in 50 to 100 mL slow IV push) to control the seizures. If you are unable to control the seizures with magnesium sulfate, consider diazepam (Valium) or another sedative. It is important to keep calcium gluconate available for use as an antidote to magnesium sulfate. Also monitor your patient closely for signs (vaginal bleeding or abdominal rigidity) of abruptio placentae or developing pulmonary edema. Transport immediately to a hospital with surgical obstetric and neonatal care availability.

Supine Hypotensive Syndrome   pp. 31–32

Supine hypotensive syndrome usually occurs in the third trimester of pregnancy. Also known as vena caval syndrome, supine hypotensive syndrome occurs when the gravid uterus compresses the inferior vena cava when the mother lies in a supine position. The patient may complain of dizziness, which results from the decrease in venous return to the right atrium and consequent lowering of the patient's blood pressure.

If there are no indications of volume depletion, such as decreased skin turgor or thirst, place the patient in the left lateral recumbent position or elevate her right hip. If there is clinical evidence of volume depletion, administer oxygen (if hypoxic) and start an IV of normal saline. Transport the patient promptly in the left lateral recumbent position.

Gestational Diabetes   p. 32

During the last 20 weeks of pregnancy, placental hormones cause an increased resistance to insulin and a decreased glucose tolerance. This causes catabolism between meals and during the night. At these times, ketones may be present in the urine because fats are metabolized more rapidly. Further, maternal glucose stores are used up, as they are the sole source of glucose to meet the energy needs of the growing fetus. This is known as the diabetogenic (diabetes-causing) effect of pregnancy. Gestational diabetes usually subsides after pregnancy. High risk is associated with maternal age (over 35), obesity, hypertension, family history of diabetes, and history of prior stillbirth.

Clinical signs and symptoms of hypoglycemia are many and varied. An abnormal mental status is the most important. Physical signs may include diaphoresis and tachycardia. Obtaining an accurate history of associated signs and symptoms, such as nausea, vomiting, abdominal pain, increased urination, or a recent infection, will allow you to ascertain whether diabetic ketoacidosis might be the cause of your patient's altered mental status. Determine the blood glucose level in addition to obtaining baseline vital signs and FHTs.

If the blood glucose level is noted to be less than 60 mg/dL, draw a red-top tube of blood and start an IV of normal saline. Next, administer 50 to 100 mL (25–50 g) of 50 percent dextrose intravenously. If the patient is conscious and able to swallow, complete glucose administration with orange juice, sugared soft drinks, or commercially available glucose pastes. If the blood glucose level is in excess of 200 mg/dL, draw a red-top tube (or the tube specified by local protocols) of blood and then establish IV access to administer 1 to 2 L of 0.9 percent sodium chloride per protocol.

Braxton-Hicks Contractions   p. 32

As early as the 13th week of gestation, the uterus contracts intermittently, thus conditioning itself for the birth process. It is also believed that these contractions enhance placental circulation. These painless, irregular contractions are known as Braxton-Hicks contractions. As the estimated date of confinement approaches, these contractions become more frequent. Ultimately, the contractions become stronger and more regular, signaling the onset of labor. It is virtually impossible to distinguish false labor from true labor in the field. Braxton-Hicks contractions do not require treatment by the paramedic aside from reassurance of the patient and, if necessary, transport for evaluation by a physician.

Preterm Labor   pp. 32–33

True labor that begins before the 38th week of gestation is called *preterm labor* and frequently requires medical intervention. A variety of maternal, fetal, or placental factors may cause this potentially life-threatening situation for the mother and fetus.

Commonly reported signs and symptoms of preterm labor include contractions that occur every 10 minutes or less, low abdominal cramping that is similar to menstrual cramps, or a sensation of pelvic pressure. Other complaints, such as low backache, changes in vaginal discharge, and abdominal cramping with or without diarrhea, may also be reported. Rupture of the membranes is confirmatory for preterm labor.

Preterm labor, especially if quite early in the pregnancy, should be stopped if possible. The process of stopping labor, or tocolysis, is frequently practiced in obstetrics. However, it is infrequently done in the field. There are three general approaches to tocolysis. The first is to sedate the patient, often with narcotics or barbiturates, thus allowing her to rest. The second approach is to administer a fluid bolus to increase the intravascular fluid volume, thus inhibiting ADH secretion from the posterior pituitary. Because oxytocin and ADH are secreted from the same area of the pituitary gland, the inhibition of ADH secretion also inhibits oxytocin release, often causing cessation of uterine contractions. Ultimately, if the above methods fail, magnesium sulfate or a beta-agonist, such as terbutaline or ritodrine, may be administered to stop labor by inhibiting uterine smooth muscle contraction.

Breech Presentation   pp. 39–40

Breech presentation is the term used to describe the situation in which either the buttocks or both feet present first. There is an increased risk for delivery trauma to the mother, as well as an increased potential for cord prolapse, cord compression, or anoxic insult for the infant. Because cesarean section is often required, delivery of the breech presentation is best accomplished at the hospital. However, if field delivery is unavoidable, position the mother with her buttocks at the edge of a firm bed. Ask her to hold her legs in a flexed position. As the infant delivers, do not pull on the infant's legs. Simply support them. Allow the entire body to be delivered with contractions while you merely continue to support the infant's body.

As the head passes the pubis, apply gentle upward traction until the mouth appears over the perineum. If the head does not deliver, and the baby begins to breathe spontaneously with its face pressed against the vaginal wall, place a gloved hand in the vagina with the palm toward the infant's face. Form a "V" with the index and middle fingers on either side of the infant's nose, and push the vaginal wall away from the infant's face to allow unrestricted respiration.

Alternatively, you may find that the shoulders, not the head, are the most difficult part to deliver. In that case, allow the body to deliver to the level of the umbilicus. Support the infant's body in your palm while gently extracting approximately 4 to 6 inches of umbilical cord. Be very careful that you do not compress the cord during this extraction. Gently rotate the infant's body so that the shoulders are now in an anterior-posterior position. Apply gentle traction to the body until the axillae become visible. Guide the infant's body upward to deliver the posterior shoulder. Then, guide the neonate downward to facilitate delivery of the anterior shoulder. Now gently ease the head through the birth canal. Continue your care of the mother and infant as you would with a normal delivery.

Prolapsed Cord   pp. 40–41

A prolapsed cord occurs when the umbilical cord precedes the fetal presenting part. This causes the cord to be compressed between the fetus and the bony pelvis, shutting off fetal circulation. If the umbilical cord is seen in the vagina, insert two fingers of a gloved hand to raise the presenting part of the fetus off the cord. At the same time, gently check the cord for pulsations, but take great care to ensure that you do not compress the cord. Place the mother in a Trendelenburg or knee-chest position. Administer oxygen (if hypoxic) and transport her immediately, with the fingers continuing to hold the presenting part off the umbilical cord. If assistance is available, apply a dressing moistened with sterile saline to the exposed cord. Do not attempt delivery, pull on the cord, or attempt to push the cord back into the vagina.

Limb Presentation   p. 41

If the baby is in a transverse lie across the uterus, an arm or leg is the presenting part protruding from the vagina. When examination of the perineum reveals a single arm or leg protruding from the birth canal, a cesarean section is necessary. Under no circumstance should you attempt a field delivery. Do not touch the extremity, pull on the extremity, or attempt to push it back into vagina. Assist the mother into a knee-chest position, as is also done when there is a prolapsed cord, and administer oxygen (if the mother is hypoxic). Provide reassurance to the mother. Transport immediately for emergency cesarean section.

©2013 Pearson Education, Inc.
Paramedic Care: Principles & Practice, Vol. 6, 4th Ed.

Multiple Births p. 42

Multiple births are fairly rare. Usually, the mother knows of, or at least suspects, the presence of more than one fetus. Multiple births should also be suspected if the mother's abdomen remains large after delivery of one baby and labor continues.

Manage this situation with the normal delivery guidelines, recognizing that you will need additional personnel and equipment to manage a multiple birth. In twin births, labor often begins earlier than expected, and the infants are generally smaller than babies born singly. Usually, one twin presents vertex and the other breech. There may be one shared placenta or two placentas. After delivery of the first baby, clamp and cut the cord. Then deliver the second baby. Because prematurity is common in multiple births, low birth weight is common and prevention of hypothermia is even more crucial.

Cephalopelvic Disproportion p. 42

Cephalopelvic disproportion occurs when the infant's head is too big to pass through the maternal pelvis easily. If cephalopelvic disproportion is not recognized and managed appropriately, fetal demise or uterine rupture may occur. There may be strong contractions for an extended period of time. On physical examination, the fetus may feel large. Also, labor generally does not progress. The fetus may be in distress, as evidenced by fetal bradycardia or meconium staining. The usual management of cephalopelvic disproportion is cesarean section. Administer oxygen to the mother (if she is hypoxic) and establish intravenous access. Transport should be immediate and rapid.

Precipitous Delivery p. 42

A precipitous delivery is a delivery that occurs after less than 3 hours of labor. This type of delivery occurs most frequently in the grand multipara and is associated with a higher-than-normal incidence of fetal trauma, tearing of the umbilical cord, or maternal lacerations. The best way to handle precipitous delivery is to be prepared. Do not turn your attention from the mother. Be ready for a rapid delivery, and attempt to control the infant's head. Once delivered, the baby may have some difficulty with temperature regulation and must be kept warm.

Shoulder Dystocia p. 42

A shoulder dystocia occurs when the infant's shoulders are larger than its head. In shoulder dystocia, labor progresses normally and the head is delivered routinely. However, immediately after the head is delivered, it retracts back into the perineum because the shoulders are trapped between the pubic symphysis and the sacrum.

If a shoulder dystocia occurs, do not pull on the infant's head. Administer oxygen to the mother (if she is hypoxic) and have her drop her buttocks off the end of the bed. Then flex her thighs upward to facilitate delivery and apply firm pressure with an open hand immediately above the pubic symphysis pubis. If delivery does not occur, transport the patient immediately.

Meconium Staining pp. 42–43

Meconium staining occurs when the fetus passes feces into the amniotic fluid. Meconium staining is often associated with prolonged labor but may be seen in term, postterm, and low-birth-weight infants. It is always indicative of a fetal hypoxic incident. Hypoxia causes an increase in fetal peristalsis along with relaxation of the anal sphincter, causing meconium to pass into the amniotic fluid. In addition to the stress that caused the incident, there is a risk of aspiration of the meconium-stained fluid. Normally the amniotic fluid is clear or possibly light-straw colored. When meconium is present, the color varies from a light yellowish-green to light green or, in the worst case, dark green, which is sometimes described as "pea soup." As a rule, the thicker and darker the color, the higher the risk of fetal morbidity.

If the meconium is thin and light colored, no further treatment is generally required and you should continue with the delivery and routine care. However, if the meconium is thick, visualize the glottis and suction the hypopharynx and trachea using an endotracheal tube until you have cleared all of the meconium from the newborn's airway. Failure to do so will cause the meconium to be pushed farther into the airway and down into the lungs during the delivery process.

Postpartum Hemorrhage p. 44

Postpartum hemorrhage is the loss of more than 500 mL of blood immediately following delivery. Assessment of the patient with should focus on the history and predisposing factors. You must rely heavily on the clinical appearance of the patient and her vital signs. Often, the uterus will feel boggy and soft on physical examination. Vaginal bleeding is usually obvious as a steady, free flow of blood. Counting the number of sanitary pads used is a good way to monitor the bleeding.

Administer oxygen (if the patient is hypoxic) and begin fundal massage. Establish at least one, preferably two, large-bore IVs of normal saline. Never attempt to force delivery of the placenta or pack the vagina with dressings. In severe cases, medical direction may request the administration of oxytocin (Pitocin). The usual dose is 10 to 20 USP units (20 mg) oxytocin in 1 liter of normal saline to run at 125 mL/hr titrated to response. If IV access cannot be obtained, an alternative therapy is to administer 10 USP units intramuscularly.

Uterine Rupture   p. 44

Uterine rupture is the actual tearing, or rupture, of the uterus. It usually occurs with the onset of labor. However, it can also occur before labor as a result of blunt abdominal trauma. The patient with uterine rupture will complain of excruciating abdominal pain and will often be in shock. On physical examination, there is often profound shock without evidence of external hemorrhage, although it is sometimes associated with vaginal bleeding. Fetal heart tones are absent. The abdomen is often tender and rigid and may exhibit rebound tenderness. It is often possible to palpate the uterus as a separate hard mass found next to the fetus.

Management is the same as for any patient in shock. Administer oxygen at high flow and high concentration. Next, establish two large-bore IVs with normal saline and begin fluid resuscitation. Monitor vital signs and fetal heart tones continuously. Transport the patient rapidly. If the fetus is still viable, the definitive treatment is cesarean section with subsequent repair or removal of the uterus.

Uterine Inversion   p. 44

Uterine inversion occurs when the uterus turns inside out after delivery and extends through the cervix. When uterine inversion occurs, the supporting ligaments and blood vessels supplying blood to the uterus are torn, usually causing profound shock. The average blood loss associated with uterine inversion ranges from 800 to 1,800 mL. Uterine inversion usually results from pulling on the umbilical cord while awaiting delivery of the placenta or from attempts to express the placenta when the uterus is relaxed.

If uterine inversion occurs, you must act quickly. First, place the patient in a supine position and begin oxygen administration (if the patient is hypoxic). Do not attempt to detach the placenta or pull on the cord. Initiate two large-bore IVs of normal saline and begin fluid resuscitation. Make one attempt to replace the uterus, using the following technique. With the palm of the hand, push the fundus of the inverted uterus toward the vagina. If this single attempt is unsuccessful, cover the uterus with towels moistened with saline and transport the patient immediately.

Pulmonary Embolism   p. 44

Pulmonary embolism is the presence of a blood clot in the pulmonary vascular system. It can occur after pregnancy, usually as a result of venous thromboembolism. It is one of the most common causes of maternal death and appears to occur more frequently following cesarean section than vaginal delivery. Pulmonary embolism may occur at any time during pregnancy. There is usually a sudden onset of severe dyspnea accompanied by sharp chest pain. Some patients also report a sense of impending doom. On physical examination, the patient may show tachycardia, tachypnea, jugular vein distention, and, in severe cases, hypotension.

Management of pulmonary embolism consists of administration of high-concentration oxygen and ventilatory support as needed. Also establish an IV of normal saline at a keep open rate. Initiate cardiac monitoring and carefully monitor the patient's vital signs and oxygen saturation while transporting her immediately.

10. **Communicate all relevant information about obstetric patients orally and in writing when transferring care to hospital personnel.**   pp. 18–44

During your classroom, clinical, and field training, you will interact and communicate with real and simulated patients, family members, bystanders, other responders, and hospital personnel. It will be important to document the time of birth in addition to the 1- and 5-minute APGAR scores. In addition to the information presented in this chapter, you will use the information from Volume 1, Chapter 9: EMS System Communications; Volume 1, Chapter 10: Documentation; and Volume 3, Chapter 3: Therapeutic Communications to effectively communicate and document assessment findings, patient management, and patient response to care. Continue to refine these skills once your training ends and you begin your career as a paramedic.

Case Study Review

Reread the case study on page 18 in Paramedic Care: Special Patients; *then, read the following discussion.*

This case study draws attention to the management of childbirth in the prehospital setting. In most cases, the role of the EMS provider in a childbirth situation is merely supportive, as often no "emergency" care is needed.

As is often the case, a great deal of information about the imminence of delivery can be obtained before physically examining the patient. This patient reveals that she has had six pregnancies, a good indicator that this delivery may proceed very quickly. The urge to move the bowels is a sign that the cervix is fully effaced and the child is moving down the birth canal. Last, when exam of the perineum displays crowning, this indicates that the cervix is fully dilated and that delivery is imminent.

Normally, preparation for delivery would entail thoroughly washing the hands and forearms before donning a gown, in addition to the gloves and goggles that were used by the EMTs. Standard Precautions for childbirth generally include draping the patient to minimize contamination of the baby during delivery. In this situation, there is no time to open the OB kit or provide for the mother's privacy.

Key EMS actions during a routine delivery are primarily supportive, but you should remain vigilant to signs of impending problems. Providing gentle support to the perineum as the delivery progresses decreases the likelihood of an explosive delivery that would cause vaginal tears and the potential for neonatal head trauma. As the head emerges from the vaginal opening, the paramedic checks to assure the umbilical cord is not wrapped around the baby's neck. Although it was once a common practice, suctioning of the nasopharynx in neonates without obvious obstruction is no longer recommended. In this scenario, the paramedics arrive in time to assist in cutting the cord, after placing clamps at 10 cm and 15 cm from the baby and cutting in between, and then drying and wrapping the baby in a warming blanket to prevent hypothermia. The mother receives fundal massage to control postpartum bleeding. Vascular access is established should fluid resuscitation become necessary. The baby is assessed and APGAR scores are identified en route to the hospital.

Childbirth is one "emergency" that almost always has a positive outcome. It is common for EMS agencies to celebrate and acknowledge such calls. Rest assured that this delivery is one the paramedic will remember for the balance of his career, even without a stork painted on his window.

Content Self-Evaluation

MULTIPLE CHOICE

_____ 1. Thickening of the uterine lining in anticipation of implantation of the fertilized egg is stimulated by
   A. estrogen.
   B. progesterone.
   C. follicle-stimulating hormone.
   D. luteinizing hormone.
   E. oxytocin.

_____ 2. All of the following are placental functions EXCEPT
   A. acting as the "organ of pregnancy."
   B. producing hormones.
   C. serving as a protective barrier.
   D. providing fertilization.
   E. providing a means of heat transfer.

3. The normal duration of pregnancy is
   A. 40 weeks.
   B. 280 days.
   C. 10 lunar months.
   D. 9 calendar months.
   E. all of the above.

4. Blood volume increases by what percentage during pregnancy?
   A. 10 percent
   B. 25 percent
   C. 30 percent
   D. 45 percent
   E. 60 percent

5. The fetus receives its oxygenated blood from the placenta by means of the
   A. umbilical vein.
   B. umbilical artery.
   C. inferior vena cava.
   D. superior vena cava.
   E. aorta.

6. Fetal circulation changes to normal circulation with the
   A. onset of labor.
   B. expulsion from the birth canal.
   C. baby's first breath.
   D. clamping of the umbilical cord.
   E. dilation and effacement of the cervix.

7. When performing a focused history on a pregnant patient, which of the following questions would be appropriate?
   A. Have you had any prenatal care?
   B. Have you had any obstetric complications in the past?
   C. When is your due date?
   D. Have you ever been pregnant before?
   E. All of the above

8. All of the following are common signs or symptoms of a predelivery emergency EXCEPT
   A. abdominal pain or trauma.
   B. vaginal bleeding or discharge.
   C. painful, deformed extremities.
   D. altered mental status or seizures.
   E. hypertension or hypotension.

9. All of the following are causes of bleeding during pregnancy EXCEPT
   A. abortion.
   B. ovarian cyst.
   C. ectopic pregnancy.
   D. placenta previa.
   E. abruptio placenta.

10. Treatment of a female patient who is 16 weeks pregnant, is complaining of cramping abdominal pain, and has bright red vaginal bleeding should include all of the following EXCEPT
    A. packing the vagina to control bleeding.
    B. treating for shock if indicated.
    C. maintaining oxygenation.
    D. providing emotional support.
    E. saving any tissue and clots for evaluation.

11. You are assessing a female patient who is 19 weeks pregnant. She is complaining of cramping abdominal pain, and has bright red vaginal bleeding. You suspect that the cause of the patient's condition is
    A. abortion.
    B. ovarian cyst.
    C. ectopic pregnancy.
    D. placenta previa.
    E. abruptio placenta.

©2013 Pearson Education, Inc.
Paramedic Care: Principles & Practice, Vol. 6, 4th Ed.

12. Pelvic inflammatory disease, use of an intrauterine device (IUD) for birth control, and tubal ligation are predisposing factors for
  A. abortion.
  B. ovarian cyst.
  C. ectopic pregnancy.
  D. placenta previa.
  E. abruptio placenta.

13. You find that your patient is 36 weeks pregnant, has an altered mental status, and is reported to have had a major motor seizure, which you suspect is due to:
  A. placenta previa.
  B. eclampsia.
  C. epilepsy.
  D. abruptio placenta.
  E. supine hypotensive syndrome.

14. You find that your patient is 35 weeks pregnant, is grossly edematous, and has an elevated blood pressure. Bystanders state the patient had a seizure. Care of this patient should include all of the following EXCEPT
  A. administering high-flow oxygen if the patient is hypoxic.
  B. protecting the patient from injury if seizures recur.
  C. administering diazepam if needed.
  D. administering magnesium sulfate per protocol.
  E. transporting on the right side to protect the airway.

15. All of the following are signs and symptoms of an imminent delivery EXCEPT
  A. the presence of crowning.
  B. contractions occurring every 1 to 2 minutes.
  C. passage of "bloody show."
  D. sensation of an urge for bowel movement.
  E. rupture of the membranes.

16. The stage of labor that begins with complete cervical dilatation and ends with the delivery of the fetus is called the dilation stage.
  A. True
  B. False

17. Your patient has just delivered a healthy baby boy. Following the delivery of the placenta, her vaginal bleeding seems to increase. Which of the following best describes what you should do to provide emergency care for this patient?
  A. Massage the uterus and position your patient on her right side.
  B. Administer oxygen and firmly massage the uterus.
  C. Massage the uterus and pack the vagina to control bleeding
  D. Administer oxygen and pack the vagina with sanitary napkins.
  E. Provide fluid resuscitation and position the patient on her right side.

18. If meconium is thick, visualize the glottis and suction the hypopharynx and trachea using an endotracheal tube until you have cleared all of the meconium from the newborn's airway.
  A. True
  B. False

19. Management of a limb presentation should include all of the following EXCEPT
  A. administrating high-flow oxygen if the mother is hypoxic.
  B. immediately transporting to the hospital.
  C. attempting to push the limb back into the vagina.
  D. positioning the mother in a knee-chest position.
  E. providing reassurance to the mother.

20. Suctioning of the nasopharynx in neonates without obvious obstruction is no longer recommended.
  A. True.
  B. False

_____ **21.** Elements of the APGAR assessment include appearance, pulse, grimace, activity, and respirations.
A. True
B. False

_____ **22.** Acrocyanosis in the neonate is always a sign of inadequate oxygenation.
A. True
B. False

_____ **23.** You have just assisted with the delivery of a baby girl. She has shallow, gasping respirations and a heart rate that is 80 beats per minute. Which of the following best describes your emergency care for this patient?
A. Administering "blow-by" oxygen and monitoring her pulse
B. Assisting ventilations with a bag-valve mask and reassessing the patient
C. Administering high-flow oxygen with a nonrebreather mask
D. Assisting ventilations with a bag-valve mask and beginning chest compressions
E. Continuing to monitor and expediting transport

_____ **24.** Shoulder dystocia is commonly associated with diabetic or obese mothers and
A. prematurity.
B. hormonal excesses.
C. postterm pregnancy.
D. hormonal deficits.
E. fetal distress.

_____ **25.** While checking for crowning, you notice the umbilical cord is presenting. All of the following are appropriate EXCEPT
A. do not pull on the cord.
B. do not attempt to push the cord back into the vagina.
C. do not attempt delivery.
D. do not place the mother in a knee-chest position.
E. do apply a moist, sterile dressing to the exposed cord.

MATCHING

Write the letter of the term in the space provided next to its definition.

A. amniotic sac
B. ovulation
C. fetus
D. placenta
E. umbilical cord

F. effacement
G. Braxton-Hicks contractions
H. parity
I. tocolysis
J. puerperium

_____ **26.** Unborn infant from the third month of pregnancy to birth

_____ **27.** Fetal lifeline, a placental extension through which the child is nourished

_____ **28.** Organ of pregnancy for the exchange of oxygen and waste products

_____ **29.** Transparent membrane forming the sac that holds the fetus

_____ **30.** Release of an egg from the ovary

_____ **31.** The time period surrounding the birth of the fetus

_____ **32.** Thinning and shortening of the cervix during labor

_____ **33.** Number of pregnancies carried to term

_____ **34.** Process of stopping labor

_____ **35.** Painless, irregular uterine contractions

©2013 Pearson Education, Inc.
Paramedic Care: Principles & Practice, Vol. 6, 4th Ed.

Special Project

Understanding the Physiological Changes of Pregnancy

Complete the following table, identifying the physiological changes of pregnancy by system and their associated EMS implications.

	Physiological Changes	**EMS Implications**
Reproductive system		
Respiratory system		
Cardiovascular system		
Gastrointestinal system		
Urinary system		
Musculoskeletal system		

Neonatology

Review of Chapter Objectives

In each chapter of the workbook, we identify the objectives and the important elements of the text content. You should review these items and refer to the pages listed if any points are not clear.

After reading this chapter, you should be able to:

1. Define key terms introduced in this chapter. pp. 47–48

Knowing and being able to apply the key terms in each chapter is critical to understanding chapter concepts. Write the list of key terms. Then write the definition of each one in your own words. Check your understanding by confirming the definitions in the text glossary. Correct any misunderstandings. Create a study aid by writing each key term on the front of an index card and the definition on the back. Use the cards to quiz yourself, or to have someone quiz you.

2. Relate the anatomy and physiology of the neonate to the assessment and management of patients one month of age and younger. pp. 48–54

Upon birth, dramatic changes occur within the newborn to prepare him extrauterine life. The respiratory system, which is essentially nonfunctional when the fetus is in the uterus, must suddenly initiate and maintain respirations. While in the uterus, fetal lung fluid fills the fetal lungs. The capillaries and arterioles of the lungs are closed. Most blood pumped by the heart bypasses the nonfunctional respiratory system by flowing through the ductus arteriosus.

Approximately one-third of fetal lung fluid is removed through compression of the chest during vaginal delivery. Under normal conditions, the newborn takes his first breath within the first few seconds after delivery. Factors that stimulate the baby's first breath include mild acidosis, initiation of stretch reflexes in the lungs, hypoxia, and hypothermia. With the first breaths, the lungs rapidly fill with air, which displaces the remaining fetal fluid.

The pulmonary arterioles and capillaries open, decreasing pulmonary vascular resistance. At this point, the resistance to blood flow in the lungs is now less than the resistance of the ductus arteriosus. Because of this pressure difference, blood flow is diverted from the ductus arteriosus to the lungs, where it picks up oxygen for transport to the peripheral tissues. Soon, there is no need for the ductus arteriosus, and it eventually closes and becomes the ligamentum arteriosum.

Many of the structures necessary for intrauterine life change following birth. The *ductus arteriosus* becomes the *ligamentum arteriosum*. The *foramen ovale* closes and becomes the *fossa ovalis*. The *ductus venosus* becomes *the ligamentus venosum*. The umbilical vein becomes the *ligamentum teres*. The umbilical arteries constrict although the proximal portions persist.

Congenital problems typically arise from a problem in fetal development. Most fetal development occurs during the first trimester of pregnancy. It is during this time that the developing fetus is most sensitive to environmental factors and substances that can affect normal development. There are a number of cardiac and noncardiac congenital anomalies that may develop.

3. **Use a process of clinical reasoning to guide and interpret the patient assessment and management process for normal and distressed neonatal patients.**   pp. 53–62

Assess the newborn immediately after birth. Make a mental note of the time of birth and then quickly obtain vital signs. The newborn's respiratory rate should average 40 to 60 breaths per minute. If respirations are not adequate or if the newborn is gasping, immediately start positive-pressure ventilation. Expect a normal heart rate of 150 to 180 beats per minute at birth, slowing to 130 to 140 beats per minute thereafter. A pulse rate of less than 100 beats per minute indicates distress and requires emergency intervention. Blood pressure will be 60 to 90 systolic and temperature will be from 36.7 to 37.8°C (98 to 100°F). Evaluate the skin color as well. Some cyanosis of the extremities is common immediately after birth. Unfortunately, cyanosis is a poor indicator of oxygen saturation in newborns.

Pulse oximetry is a better indicator of oxygen saturation. It is important to remember that neonatal oxygen saturations do not reach normal levels until approximately 10 minutes after birth. They are initially in the 70 to 80 percent range. Supplemental oxygen should be provided only in cases in which oxygen saturation levels are below normal. If needed, administer only enough oxygen to maintain the normal oxygen saturation.

Ideally, an APGAR score should be assigned at 1 and 5 minutes after birth. However, if the newborn is not breathing, do not withhold resuscitation in order to determine the APGAR score. The APGAR scoring system helps distinguish between newborns who need only routine care and those who need greater assistance. The system also predicts long-term survival. APGAR scoring consists of: appearance, pulse rate, grimace, activity, and respiratory effort. A score of 0, 1, or 2 is given for each of the parameters. The minimum total score is 0 and the maximum is 10. A score of 7 to 10 indicates an active and vigorous newborn who requires only routine care. A score of 4 to 6 indicates a moderately distressed newborn who requires oxygenation and stimulation. Severely distressed newborns, those with APGAR scores of less than 4, require immediate resuscitation.

Management of a normal newborn focuses on establishing the airway, preventing heat loss, and cutting the umbilical cord. Management of the distressed newborn follows the inverted pyramid. Step 1 involves drying, warming, positioning, suctioning, and tactile stimulation. Step 2 involves ventilation. Step 3 involves supplemental oxygen. Step 4 involves chest compressions. Step 5 involves medications and fluids.

4. **Adapt the scene size-up, primary assessment, patient history, secondary assessment, and use of monitoring technology to meet the needs of normal and distressed neonatal patients.**   pp. 53–62

The initial care of a newborn follows the same priorities as care for all patients. Complete the primary assessment first. Correct any problems detected during the primary assessment before proceeding to the next step. The vast majority of term newborns, approximately 80 percent, will require no resuscitation beyond suctioning of the airway, mild stimulation, and maintenance of body temperature by drying and warming with blankets.

Bulb suctioning during delivery and following delivery was once a common practice. However, it has been found to be relatively ineffective and can actually cause neonatal bradycardia. It is no longer recommended. Thus, if the amniotic fluid is clear, suctioning (either bulb or otherwise) is indicated only in babies with an obstruction to spontaneous breathing or who require positive-pressure ventilation. If meconium is present, especially thick meconium, consider endotracheal intubation and endotracheal suctioning of nonvigorous neonates.

Drying and tactile stimulation usually produces enough stimulation to initiate respirations in most newborns. If the newborn does not cry immediately, stimulate him by flicking the soles of his feet or gently rubbing his back. Do not spank or vigorously rub a newborn baby. Heat loss can be a life-threatening condition in newborns. Cold infants quickly become distressed infants. Heat loss occurs through evaporation, convection, conduction, and radiation. Most heat loss in newborns results from evaporation. The newborn comes into the world wet, and the amniotic fluid quickly evaporates.

After you have stabilized the newborn's airway and minimized heat loss, clamp and cut the umbilical cord. You can prevent over- and undertransfusion of blood by maintaining the baby at the same level as the mother's vagina, as previously described. Do not "milk" or strip the umbilical cord. Apply the umbilical clamps within 30 to 45 seconds after birth. Place the first clamp approximately

10 cm (4 inches) from the newborn. Place the second clamp about 5 cm (2 inches) farther away than the first. Then cut the cord between the two clamps. After the cord is cut, inspect it periodically to make sure there is no additional bleeding.

The most common problem experienced by newborns during the first minutes of life is ventilation. For this reason, resuscitation usually consists of ventilation and, if needed, oxygenation. Except in special situations, the use of IV fluids, drugs, or cardiac equipment is usually not indicated. The most important procedures include suctioning, drying, and stimulating the distressed newborn.

Of the vital signs, fetal heart rate is the most important indicator of neonatal distress. The newborn has a relatively fixed stroke volume. Thus, cardiac output depends more on heart rate than on stroke volume. Bradycardia, as caused by hypoxia, results in decreased cardiac output and, ultimately, poor perfusion. A pulse rate of less than 60 beats per minute in a distressed newborn should be treated with chest compressions. In distressed newborns, monitor the heart rate manually. Do not depend on external electronic monitors.

Resuscitation of the newborn follows an inverted pyramid. As this pyramid indicates, most distressed newborns respond to relatively simple maneuvers. Few require cardiopulmonary resuscitation (CPR) or advanced life-support measures. Step 1 involves drying, warming, positioning, suctioning, and tactile stimulation. Step 2 involves ventilation. Step 3 involves supplemental oxygen. Step 4 involves chest compressions. Step 5 involves medications and fluids.

5. Demonstrate concern for the psychosocial needs of the parents of normal and distressed neonates. pp. 53–62

As you learned in the previous chapter, most births occur without complications. Whether you are caring for a newborn requiring only minimal interventions such as drying and stimulating or a distressed newborn requiring more extensive care such as cardiopulmonary resuscitation and medications, your professionalism and compassion toward the patient and parents or caregivers will be remembered and appreciated.

6. Recognize specific problems in neonates, including meconium aspiration, apnea, respiratory distress, cyanosis, cardiac arrest, bradycardia, prematurity, seizures, fever, hypothermia, hypoglycemia, dehydration, and birth injuries.

Meconium-Stained Amniotic Fluid
p. 62

Meconium-stained amniotic fluid occurs in approximately 10 to 15 percent of deliveries, mostly in post-term or small-for-gestational-age newborns. Meconium aspiration accounts for a significant proportion of neonatal deaths. Fetal distress and hypoxia can cause meconium to be passed into the amniotic fluid. Either in utero or more often with the first breath, thick meconium is aspirated into the lungs, resulting in small-airway obstruction and aspiration pneumonia.

Apnea
p. 63

This condition is a common finding in the preterm infant or infants weighing less than 1,500 grams (3 pounds, 5 ounces), infants exposed to drugs, or infants born after prolonged or difficult labor and delivery. Typically, the infant fails to breathe spontaneously after stimulation, or the infant experiences respiratory pauses of more than 20 seconds. Apnea can be due to hypoxia, hypothermia, narcotic or central nervous system depressants, weakness of the respiratory muscles, septicemia, metabolic disorders, or central nervous system disorders.

Diaphragmatic Hernia
p. 63

Diaphragmatic hernias rarely occur. They are seen in approximately 1 out of every 2,200 live births. When they do appear, the herniation takes place most often in the posterolateral segments of the diaphragm, and most commonly (90 percent) on the left side. The defect is caused by the failure of the pleuroperitoneal canal to close completely. The survival rate for infants who require mechanical ventilation in the first 18 to 24 hours is approximately 50 percent. However, if there is no respiratory distress in the first 24 hours of life, the survival rate approaches 100 percent.

Protrusion of abdominal viscera through the hernia into the thoracic cavity occurs in varying degrees. In severe cases, the stomach and a large part of the intestines and the spleen, liver, and kidneys displace the lungs and heart to the opposite side. The lung on the affected side is compressed, causing diminished total lung volume.

Bradycardia   pp. 63–64
Bradycardia is most commonly caused by hypoxia in newborns. However, bradycardia may also be caused by several other factors, including increased intracranial pressure, hypothyroidism, or acidosis. In cases of hypoxia, the infant experiences minimal risk if the hypoxia is corrected quickly.

Prematurity   p. 64
A premature newborn is an infant born prior to 37 weeks of gestation or with weight ranging from 0.6 to 2.2 kg (1 pound, 5 ounces, to 4 pounds, 13 ounces). Mortality decreases weekly with gestation beyond the onset of fetal viability. Premature newborns are at greater risk of respiratory suppression, head or brain injury caused by hypoxemia, changes in blood pressure, intraventricular hemorrhage, and fluctuations in serum osmolarity. They are also more susceptible to hypothermia than full-term newborns.

Respiratory Distress/Cyanosis   p. 64
Prematurity is the single most common factor causing respiratory distress and cyanosis in the newborn. The problem occurs most frequently in infants weighing less than 1,200 grams (2 pounds, 10 ounces) and who are born at less than 30 weeks of gestation. Premature infants have an immature central respiratory control center and are easily affected by environmental or metabolic changes. Contributing factors to respiratory distress include lung or heart disease, central nervous system disorders, meconium aspiration, metabolic problems, obstruction of the nasal passages, shock and sepsis, and diaphragmatic hernia.

Hypovolemia   pp. 65–66
Hypovolemia is the leading cause of shock in newborns. It may result from dehydration, hemorrhage, or third-spacing of fluids. Dehydration is by far the most common cause.

Seizures   p. 65
Neonatal seizures differ from seizures in a child or an adult, because generalized tonic-clonic convulsions rarely occur in the first month of life. Types of seizures in the neonate include:

- Subtle seizures—consist of chewing motions and excessive salivation, blinking, sucking, swimming movements of the arms, pedaling movements of the legs, apnea, and color changes.
- Tonic seizures—characterized by rigid posturing of the extremities and trunk; sometimes associated with fixed deviation of the eyes.
- Focal clonic seizures—consist of rhythmic twitching of muscle groups, particularly in the extremities and face.
- Multifocal seizures—exhibit signs similar to focal clonic seizures, except multiple muscle groups are involved, and clonic activity randomly migrates.
- Myoclonic seizures—characterized by brief focal or generalized jerks of the extremities or parts of the body that tend to involve distal muscle groups.

The causes of neonatal seizures include sepsis, fever, hypoglycemia, hypoxic-ischemic encephalopathy, metabolic disturbances, meningitis, development abnormalities, and drug withdrawal.

Fever   p. 65
Neonates do not develop fever as easily as older children. Therefore, any fever in a neonate requires extensive evaluation because it is more likely to be caused by a life-threatening condition such as pneumonia, sepsis, or meningitis. In fact, fever may be the only sign of meningitis in a neonate. Because of their immature development, neonates do not exhibit the classic symptoms such as a stiff neck.

©2013 Pearson Education, Inc.
Paramedic Care: Principles & Practice, Vol. 6, 4th Ed.

Hypothermia
pp. 65–66

Hypothermia presents a common and life-threatening condition for newborns. The increased surface-to-volume relationship in newborns makes them extremely sensitive to environmental temperatures, especially right after delivery when they are wet. In treating hypothermia—a body temperature below 35°C (95°F)—try to control the loss of heat through evaporation, conduction, convection, and radiation. Also remember that hypothermia can be an indicator of sepsis in the newborn. Regardless of the cause, the increase in the metabolic demands can produce a variety of related conditions, including metabolic acidosis, pulmonary hypertension, and hypoxemia.

Hypoglycemia
p. 66

Newborns are the only age group that can develop severe hypoglycemia and not have diabetes mellitus. Hypoglycemia may be caused by inadequate glucose intake or increased glucose utilization. Stress and other factors can also cause the blood sugar to fall, sometimes to a critical level. Hypoglycemia is more common in premature or small-for-gestational-age (SGA) infants, the smaller twin, and newborns of a diabetic mother, because these infants often have decreased glycogen stores. Hypoglycemia can also develop as a result of increased glucose utilization. Causes include respiratory illnesses, hypothermia, toxemia, central nervous system (CNS) hemorrhage, asphyxia, meningitis, and sepsis. In an older infant, hypoglycemia may be caused by an inadequate glucose intake or increased utilization of glucose. Infants receiving glucose infusions can develop hypoglycemia if the infusion is suddenly stopped.

Vomiting/Diarrhea
pp. 66–67

Vomiting in a neonate may result from a variety of causes and rarely presents as an isolated symptom. Vomiting—the forceful ejection of stomach contents—rarely occurs during the first weeks of life and may be confused with regurgitation or "spitting up." Causes of vomiting include a tracheoesophageal fistula, an upper gastrointestinal obstruction, increased intracranial pressure, or an infection. Vomit containing dark blood signals a life-threatening illness. Keep in mind, however, that vomiting of mucus, which may occasionally be streaked with blood, in the first few hours after birth is not uncommon.

Diarrhea can cause severe dehydration and electrolyte imbalances in the neonate. Normally five to six stools per day can be expected, especially in breast-fed infants. Causes of diarrhea in a neonate include bacterial or viral infection, gastroenteritis, lactose intolerance, phototherapy, neonatal abstinence syndrome (NAS), thyrotoxicosis, and cystic fibrosis. In managing an infant with diarrhea, remember Standard Precautions.

Birth Injuries
p. 67

A birth injury occurs in an estimated 2 to 7 of every 1,000 live births in the United States. About 5 to 8 of every 100,000 infants die of birth trauma and 25 of every 100,000 die of anoxic injuries. These injuries account for 2 to 3 percent of infant deaths. Risk factors for birth injury include prematurity, postmaturity, cephalopelvic disproportion, prolonged labor, breech presentation, explosive delivery, shoulder dystocia, and a diabetic mother.

Birth injuries can take various forms. Cranial injuries may include molding of the head and overriding of the parietal bones, erythema, abrasions, ecchymosis, subcutaneous fat necrosis, subconjunctival and retinal hemorrhage, subperiosteal hemorrhage, and fracture of the skull. Often the infant will develop a large scalp hematoma, called a caput succedaneum, during the birth process, but this condition will usually resolve over a week's time. Other birth injuries include peripheral nerve injury, injury to the liver, rupture of the spleen, adrenal hemorrhage, fractures of the clavicle or extremities, and hypoxia-ischemia.

Cardiac Arrest
pp. 67–68

The incidence of neonatal cardiac arrest is related primarily to hypoxia. The condition can be caused by primary or secondary apnea, bradycardia, persistent fetal circulation, or pulmonary hypertension. Unless appropriate interventions are initiated immediately, the outcome is poor.

Risk factors for cardiac arrest in newborns include bradycardia, intrauterine asphyxia, prematurity, drugs administered to or taken by the mother, congenital neuromuscular diseases, congenital malformations, and intrapartum hypoxemia. Assessment findings may include peripheral cyanosis, inadequate respiratory effort, and ineffective or absent heart rate.

7. **Relate the pathophysiology of specific neonatal problems to the priorities of patient assessment and management.**

Meconium-Stained Amniotic Fluid   p. 62

The infant may have respiratory distress within the first hours, or even the first minutes, of life, as evidenced by tachypnea, retraction, grunting, and cyanosis in severely affected newborns. The partial obstruction of some airways may lead to a pneumothorax.

Infants born through thin meconium may not require treatment if they are vigorous (strong respiratory efforts, good muscle tone, and heart rate > 100 per minute), but nonvigorous infants born through thick, particulate (pea-soup), meconium-stained fluid should be intubated immediately, prior to the first ventilation. Before stimulating such infants to breathe, apply suction with a meconium aspirator attached to an endotracheal (ET) tube. Connect to suction at 100 cm H_2O or less to remove meconium from the airway. Withdraw the ET tube as suction is applied. It may be necessary to repeat this procedure to clear the airway. The patient should then be taken to a facility that can manage a high-risk neonate.

Apnea   p. 63

Management begins with tactile stimulation, followed by bag-valve-mask ventilation, with the pop-off valve disabled. If the infant does not breathe on his own, or if the heart rate is less than 60 with adequate ventilation and chest compressions, perform tracheal intubation with direct visualization. Generally, neonatal naloxone is no longer recommended. Throughout the treatment, keep the infant warm to prevent hypothermia.

Diaphragmatic Hernia   p. 63

Assessment findings may include little to severe distress present from birth, dyspnea and cyanosis unresponsive to ventilations, small and flat (scaphoid) abdomen, bowel sounds in the chest, and heart sounds displaced to the right. As soon as you suspect a diaphragmatic hernia, position the infant with his head and thorax higher than the abdomen and feet. Place a nasogastric or orogastric tube and apply low, intermittent suctioning. This will decrease the entrapment of air and fluid within the herniated viscera and will reduce the degree of ventilatory compromise. Do not use bag-valve-mask ventilation, which can worsen this condition by causing gastric distention. If necessary, cautiously administer positive-pressure ventilation through an endotracheal tube. This condition usually requires surgical repair. Explain the possible need for surgery to parents, assuring them that their newborn child will be transported quickly to the facility best able to handle this procedure.

Bradycardia   pp. 63–64

In providing treatment, follow the procedures in the inverted pyramid. Resist the inclination to treat the bradycardia with pharmacological measures alone. Keep the newborn warm and transport to the nearest facility.

Prematurity   p. 64

The degree of immaturity determines the physical characteristics of a premature newborn. Premature newborns often appear to have a larger head relative to body size. They may have large trunks and short extremities, transparent skin, and few wrinkles.

Prematurity should not be a factor in short-term treatment. Resuscitation should be attempted if there is any sign of life, and the measures of resuscitation should be the same as those for newborns of normal weight and maturity. Maintain a patent airway and avoid potential aspiration of gastric contents.

Respiratory Distress/Cyanosis   p. 64

Expect the following assessment findings: tachypnea, paradoxical breathing, intercostal retractions, nasal flaring, and expiratory grunt.

In providing treatment, follow the inverted pyramid, paying particular attention to airway and ventilation. Suction as needed and provide high-concentration oxygen. If prolonged ventilation will be required, consider placing an endotracheal tube. Perform chest compressions, if indicated. Consider dextrose ($D_{10}W$ or $D_{25}W$) solution if the newborn is hypoglycemic. Maintain body temperature and transport to the most appropriate facility.

©2013 Pearson Education, Inc.
Paramedic Care: Principles & Practice, Vol. 6, 4th Ed.

Hypovolemia

pp. 64–65

Signs of hypovolemia include pale color, cool skin, diminished peripheral pulses, delayed capillary refill despite normal ambient temperature, mental status changes, and diminished urination (oliguria).

When you observe these signs, administer a fluid bolus and assess the infant's response. If signs of shock continue, administer a second bolus. Additional boluses should be infused as indicated by repeated assessments. A hypovolemic infant may often need 40 to 60 mL/kg of fluid during the first hour of resuscitation. Fluid bolus resuscitation consists of 10 mL/kg of an isotonic crystalloid solution, such as Ringer's lactate or normal saline. Administer the bolus over 5 to 10 minutes as soon as intravascular or intraosseous access is obtained. Do not use solutions containing dextrose, because they can produce hypokalemia or worsen ischemic brain injury. Avoid giving volume expanders too rapidly, as rapid infusion of large volumes of fluid has been associated with brain (intraventricular) hemorrhage.

Seizures

p. 65

Assessment findings of seizures include decreased level of consciousness and seizure activity as already described. Treatment focuses on airway management, oxygen saturation, and administration of an anticonvulsant. You might administer a benzodiazepine (usually lorazepam) for status epilepticus or dextrose ($D_{10}W$ or $D_{25}W$) for hypoglycemia.

Fever

p. 65

Assessment findings of a fever include changes in mental status (irritability or somnolence), decreased feeding, skin warm to the touch, and rashes or petechiae. Term infants may form beads of sweat on their brows, but not on the rest of their bodies. Premature infants, on the other hand, will have no visible sweat at all.

Treatment of the neonate with a fever will, for the most part, be limited to ensuring a patent airway and adequate ventilation. Do not use cold packs, which may drop the temperature too quickly and may also cause seizures. If the newborn becomes bradycardic, provide chest compressions.

Hypothermia

pp. 65–66

In assessing hypothermic newborns, remember that they do not shiver. Instead, expect the following findings: pale color, skin cool to the touch (especially in the extremities), acrocyanosis, respiratory distress, possible apnea, bradycardia, central cyanosis, initial irritability, and lethargy in later stages. Management focuses on ensuring adequate ventilations and oxygenation. Chest compressions may be necessary with bradycardia.

Hypoglycemia

p. 66

Infants with hypoglycemia may be asymptomatic or they may exhibit symptoms such as apnea, color changes, respiratory distress, lethargy, seizures, acidosis, and poor myocardial contractility. Assessment findings may include twitching or seizures, limpness, lethargy, eye-rolling, high-pitched cry, apnea, irregular respirations, and possible cyanosis. Treatment begins with management of airway and ventilations. Administer chest compressions, if needed. With medical direction, administer dextrose ($D_{10}W$ or $D_{25}W$).

Vomiting/Diarrhea

pp. 66–67

Assessment findings may include distended stomach, signs of infection, increased intracranial pressure, or drug withdrawal. Because vomitus can be aspirated, management considerations focus on ensuring a patent airway to prevent aspiration. If you detect respiratory difficulty, suction or clear the vomitus from the airway and oxygenate as needed. Fluid administration may be necessary to prevent dehydration. Remember that, as with older patients, vagal stimulation may cause bradycardia in the neonate.

Management consists of maintenance of airway and ventilations, adequate oxygenation, and chest compressions, if indicated. With medical direction, administer fluid therapy to prevent or treat dehydration.

Birth Injuries

p. 67

Assessment findings may include diffuse (sometimes ecchymotic) edematous swelling of soft tissues around the scalp, paralysis below the level of the spinal cord injury, paralysis of the upper arm with or without paralysis of the forearm, diaphragmatic paralysis, movement on only one side of the face when crying, inability to move the arm freely on the side of the fractured clavicle, lack of spontaneous movement of the affected extremity, hypoxia, and shock. Management of a newborn who has suffered a birth injury is specific to the injury but always centers on protection of the airway, provision of adequate ventilation, and chest compressions, if necessary.

Cardiac Arrest   pp. 67–68

In managing the neonatal cardiac arrest, follow the inverted pyramid for resuscitation and administer drugs or fluids according to medical direction. Postarrest management involves maintenance of the infant's body temperature, prompt transport to the appropriate facility, and delicate handling of the parents or caregivers.

8. **Communicate relevant patient information orally and in writing when transferring care of the neonatal patient to hospital personnel.**   pp. 48–68

During your classroom, clinical, and field training, you will interact and communicate with real and simulated patients, family members, bystanders, other responders, and hospital personnel. In addition to the information presented in this chapter, you will use the information from Volume 1, Chapter 9: EMS System Communications; Volume 1, Chapter 10: Documentation; and Volume 3, Chapter 3: Therapeutic Communications to effectively communicate and document assessment findings, patient management, and patient response to care. Continue to refine these skills once your training ends and you begin your career as a paramedic.

Case Study Review

Reread the case study on page 48 in Paramedic Care: Special Patients; *then, read the following discussion.*
This case study draws attention to one of the complications that may occur in a prehospital delivery of a newborn.

In this case, you arrive on scene to attend one patient, a woman who has just gone into labor, and quickly find yourself managing a second patient—a newly born infant who remains blue and limp, even after quickly drying the infant and wrapping her in a dry blanket, reducing the life-threatening risk of hypothermia. The situation can be highly stressful, especially with the two parents nearby. You recall the steps in the inverted pyramid for resuscitating a distressed newborn. As you prepare to suction, you remember that you will also need to apply tactile stimulation, either by flicking the soles of the newborn's feet or by gently rubbing her back.

When the baby does not "pink up," many thoughts probably run through your mind. You know, for example, that a prolonged lack of oxygen can cause permanent brain damage—and death. Use of the APGAR score is out of the question. You must immediately provide the patient with oxygen. Again following the inverted pyramid, you administer supplemental oxygen (preferably warmed and humidified) using the blow-by method. The baby remains blue and limp, so you begin positive-pressure ventilation with a bag-valve-mask unit, the device of choice. Perhaps you also depress the pop-off valve to deactivate it and ensure adequate ventilation.

Because the baby "pinks up" and begins to cry, you do not have to initiate endotracheal intubation or chest compressions. You still use the pulse oximeter to ensure adequate oxygen saturation. In preparing the newborn for transport, keep in mind the risk of hypothermia and cover the baby's head to prevent unnecessary heat loss. En route to the hospital, with the baby receiving blow-by oxygen, you finally compute the APGAR score. You come up with a 9—1 point below the maximum!

Remember, too, that the mother is a patient as well and needs a physical assessment and frequent monitoring. Your calm, professional conduct throughout the call helped reassure the parents—the two other people in your care—of their daughter's safety. In recognition of a job well done, they name her after you.

©2013 Pearson Education, Inc.
Paramedic Care: Principles & Practice, Vol. 6, 4th Ed.

Content Self-Evaluation

MULTIPLE CHOICE

_____ 1. Examples of antepartum factors indicating possible complications in newborns include multiple gestation and

    A. premature labor.
    B. inadequate prenatal care.
    C. abnormal presentation.
    D. prolapsed cord.
    E. prolonged labor.

_____ 2. Examples of intrapartum factors indicating possible complications in newborns include the mother's use of narcotics within 4 hours of delivery and

    A. meconium-stained amniotic fluid.
    B. postterm gestation.
    C. a mother under 16 years old.
    D. toxemia or diabetes.
    E. a mother over 35 years old.

_____ 3. When the fetus is in the uterus, the respiratory system is

    A. working at a very rapid speed.
    B. working at a very slow speed.
    C. essentially nonfunctional.
    D. essentially functional.
    E. flushed with meconium.

_____ 4. Factors that stimulate the baby's first breath include

    A. mild acidosis.
    B. hypoxia.
    C. hypothermia.
    D. initiation of stretch reflexes in the lungs.
    E. all of the above.

_____ 5. Persistent fetal circulation is a condition in which the

    A. ductus arteriosus remains closed.
    B. ductus arteriosus reopens.
    C. pulmonary vascular bed dilates.
    D. both A and C.
    E. both B and C.

_____ 6. During secondary apnea, the infant takes several last deep, gasping respirations.

    A. True
    B. False

_____ 7. Most of the fetal development that could lead to congenital problems occurs during the

    A. first trimester.
    B. second trimester.
    C. third trimester.
    D. onset of labor.
    E. intrapartum period.

_____ 8. Some infants are born with a defect in their spinal cord. In some cases, the spinal cord and associated structures may be exposed. This abnormality is called diaphragmatic hernia.

    A. True
    B. False

_____ 9. A congenital hernia of the umbilicus found in the neonate is called

    A. a choanal atresia.
    B. Pierre Robin syndrome.
    C. spina bifida.
    D. a meningomyelocele.
    E. an omphalocele.

_____ 10. A congenital condition characterized by a small jaw combined with a cleft palate, downward displacement of the tongue, and an absent gag reflex is called

    A. cleft lip.
    B. an omphalocele.
    C. cleft palate.
    D. Pierre Robin syndrome.
    E. a choanal atresia.

_____ 11. The normal newborn respiratory rate is _____ breaths per minute.
   A. 10 to 30
   B. 20 to 50
   C. 30 to 60
   D. 40 to 70
   E. 60 to 90

_____ 12. The normal newborn heart rate is _____ beats per minute.
   A. 60 to 100
   B. 80 to 120
   C. 100 to 180
   D. 120 to 180
   E. 140 to 180

_____ 13. The normal newborn systolic blood pressure is _____ mmHg.
   A. 40 to 80
   B. 60 to 90
   C. 80 to 100
   D. 100 to 120
   E. 120 to 140

_____ 14. If the newborn is not breathing, do NOT withhold resuscitation in order to determine the APGAR score.
   A. True
   B. False

_____ 15. The G in APGAR stands for
   A. gravida.
   B. gestation.
   C. grimace.
   D. gray tone.
   E. none of the above.

_____ 16. Bulb suctioning during delivery and following delivery is no longer recommended due to ineffectiveness and the possibility of causing
   A. bradycardia.
   B. tachycardia.
   C. bradypnea.
   D. tachypnea.
   E. none of the above.

_____ 17. If the amniotic fluid is clear, suctioning is indicated only in babies with an obstruction to spontaneous breathing or who require positive-pressure ventilation.
   A. True
   B. False

_____ 18. Loss of heat by the newborn can occur through
   A. evaporation.
   B. convection.
   C. conduction.
   D. radiation.
   E. all of the above.

_____ 19. Immediately after birth, the newborn's core temperature can drop 4 degrees or more from his birth temperature.
   A. True
   B. False

_____ 20. Prior to cutting the umbilical cord, it should not be "milked," as this can cause
   A. polycythemia.
   B. anemia.
   C. hyperbilirubinemia.
   D. hemophilia.
   E. both A and C.

_____ 21. An increase in the level of bilirubin in the blood can cause
   A. jaundice.
   B. pallor.
   C. cyanosis.
   D. flushing.
   E. anemia.

_____ 22. The most important indicator of neonatal distress is the fetal respiratory rate.
   A. True
   B. False

©2013 Pearson Education, Inc.
Paramedic Care: Principles & Practice, Vol. 6, 4th Ed.

23. EMS units should contain all of the following equipment in their neonatal resuscitation kit, EXCEPT
   A. a meconium aspirator.
   B. a laryngoscope with size 3 and 4 blades.
   C. a device to secure the endotracheal tube.
   D. an umbilical catheter and 10-mL syringe.
   E. epinephrine 1:10,000 and 1:1,000.

24. In following the inverted pyramid of neonatal resuscitation, which would be done first?
   A. Intubation
   B. Bag-valve-mask ventilations
   C. Chest compressions
   D. Drying and warming
   E. Administration of medications

25. In distressed newborns, monitor the heart rate with external electronic monitors.
   A. True
   B. False

26. Insertion of an endotracheal tube is recommended when prolonged ventilation of a newborn will be required.
   A. True
   B. False

27. Initiate chest compressions in the newborn with which of the following?
   A. Heart rate greater than 100
   B. Heart rate less than 60
   C. No respirations
   D. Heart rate between 60 and 80 that does not improve
   E. Both A and D

28. The proper size of catheter used to cannulate the umbilical vein is
   A. 14 ga.
   B. 22 ga.
   C. 10 fr.
   D. 5 fr.
   E. 2 fr.

29. The narcotic antagonist naloxone (Narcan) is NOT indicated in neonatal resuscitation.
   A. True
   B. False

30. Remove the endotracheal tube as you suction the neonate with possible meconium aspiration.
   A. True
   B. False

31. Which of the following is NOT a causative factor for apnea?
   A. CNS depressants
   B. Caffeine
   C. Septicemia
   D. Metabolic disorders
   E. Weak respiratory muscles

32. The most common cause of bradycardia in the newborn is
   A. increasing intracranial pressure.
   B. narcotic overdose.
   C. cerebral palsy.
   D. hypoxia.
   E. congenital cardiac problems.

33. The initial bolus of fluid for the dehydrated neonate is
   A. 10 mL/kg.
   B. 20 mL/kg.
   C. 40 mL/kg.
   D. 60 mL/kg.
   E. none of the above.

34. In assessing hypothermic newborns, remember that they do not shiver.
   A. True
   B. False

_____ **35.** Hypoglycemia is only associated with severe diabetes mellitus in the newborn.
  A. True
  B. False

Special Project

The APGAR Scale

The APGAR scoring system will help you distinguish between newborns who need only routine care and those who needed greater assistance. To gain practice in using this system, complete the following exercises.

Part I

You have just assisted in the delivery of a newborn. Your quick assessment reveals a blue baby with very slow movement of the extremities. Your initial vital signs indicate a slow respiratory rate and a heart rate around 80 to 90 beats per minute. The infant seems distressed but does not cry when touched. Complete the first 1-minute APGAR score for this infant using the following chart.

The APGAR Score					
				Score	
Sign	0	1	2	1 min.	5 min.
Appearance (Skin color)	Blue, pale	Body pink, extremities blue	Completely pink		
Pulse Rate (Heart rate)	Absent	Below 100	Above 100		
Grimace (Irritability)	No response	Grimace	Cries		
Activity (Muscle tone)	Limp	Some flexion of extremities	Active motion		
Respiratory Effort	Absent	Slow and irregular	Strong cry		
			TOTAL SCORE =		

Part II

You have begun to follow the inverted pyramid by drying, warming, positioning, suctioning, and providing tactile stimulation to the newborn. Based upon the inverted pyramid, what would be the next steps if the infant does not "pink up"? Indicate these steps, in the correct order, on the following incomplete diagram.

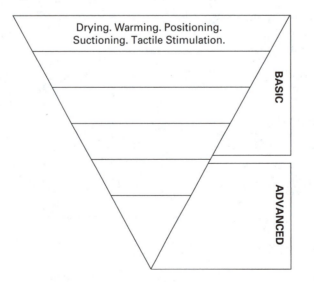

©2013 Pearson Education, Inc.
Paramedic Care: Principles & Practice, Vol. 6, 4th Ed.

Part III

Fortunately, the stimulation that you provided has been helpful. At this time, both the family and your crew feel immense relief as the infant begins to cry and thrash about. A quick assessment of the vitals reveals a pulse rate well over 100 beats per minute. The infant's body is now pink, but the extremities are still a bit blue. Recalculate the APGAR score, using the chart in Part I, now that 5 minutes have quickly gone by.

4 Pediatrics

Review of Chapter Objectives

In each chapter of the workbook, we identify the objectives and the important elements of the text content. You should review these items and refer to the pages listed if any points are not clear.

After reading this chapter, you should be able to:

1. Define key terms introduced in this chapter. p. 71

Knowing and being able to apply the key terms in each chapter is critical to understanding chapter concepts. Write the list of key terms. Then write the definition of each one in your own words. Check your understanding by confirming the definitions in the text glossary. Correct any misunderstandings. Create a study aid by writing each key term on the front of an index card and the definition on the back. Use the cards to quiz yourself, or to have someone quiz you.

2. Describe the roles of paramedics in pediatric illness and injury prevention and in the management of ill and injured children. pp. 72–73

When considering the reduction of pediatric morbidity and mortality, your role as a paramedic centers around two key concepts. First, you must realize that pediatric injuries have become a major health concern. Second, you should remember that children are at a higher risk of injury than adults and that they are more likely to be adversely affected by the injuries that they suffer.

Numerous factors account for the high pediatric injury rates. Some factors, such as geography and weather, cannot be altered. However, other factors, particularly dangers within the home and community, can be eliminated or minimized. As health care professionals, we must all get involved in identifying and implementing methods and mechanisms that prevent injuries to infants and children. Those of us who deliver prehospital care must do more than simply enter the picture after an injury has taken place. It is important that the paramedic be familiar with the many aspects of disease and disease processes that are unique to children, because early intervention is often the key to reduced morbidity and mortality.

3. Formulate a plan for becoming and remaining proficient in assessing and managing pediatric patients. pp. 72–73

Your role in improving the health care offered to pediatric patients begins with your own training. Because you will encounter pediatric patients less frequently than adult patients, you have a professional responsibility to maintain and improve upon your pediatric knowledge, particularly your clinical skills. Continuing education programs include Pediatric Advanced Life Support (PALS), Pediatric Education for Paramedic Professionals (PEPP), Advanced Pediatric Life Support (APLS), Prehospital Pediatric Care (PPC), and regional conferences and seminars that are designed to increase your knowledge of pediatric care.

You can further enhance your clinical skills by spending time in pediatric emergency departments, pediatric hospitals, or pediatric departments in local hospitals. You might also visit the offices of pediatricians or talk with pediatric nurse practitioners who provide primary health care to children.

It is important to remember that the less frequently a skill is used, the more frequently it should be practiced. Certain ALS skills can be lifesaving when properly applied. Thus, it is incumbent on each paramedic to realize that pediatric ALS skills will be needed infrequently. When they are needed, however, they must be applied competently.

4. **Relate the developmental, anatomic, and physiologic differences of children of various ages to adaptations in communication, assessment, and management of pediatric patients.**

Children are broken into age groups because they differ in terms of anatomical, physiological, growth, and developmental characteristics. The following are some of the differences:

Newborns (First Hours After Birth) p. 74

Although the terms *newborn* and *neonate* are often used interchangeably, *newborn* refers to a baby in the first hours of extrauterine life. The term *neonate* describes infants from birth to 1 month of age. The method most frequently used to assess newborns is the APGAR scoring system, which was described in Chapter 3. Resuscitation of the newborn generally follows the inverted pyramid described in Chapter 3 and the guidelines established in the Neonatal Advanced Life Support (NALS) curriculum.

Neonates (Birth to 1 Month) p. 74

The neonate, as just noted and as described in Chapter 3, is an infant up to 1 month of age. This is a major stage of development. Soon after birth, the neonate typically loses up to 10 percent of his birth weight as he adjusts to extrauterine life. This lost weight, however, is ordinarily recovered within 10 days. Gestational age affects early growth. Children born at term (40 weeks) should follow accepted developmental guidelines. Infants born prematurely will not be as developed, both neurologically and physically, as their term counterparts.

The neonatal stage of development centers on reflexes. The neonate's personality also begins to form. The infant is close to the mother and may stare at faces and smile. The mother, and occasionally the father, can comfort and quiet the child. Common illnesses in this age group include jaundice, vomiting, and respiratory distress. Serious illnesses, such as meningitis, are difficult to distinguish from minor illnesses in neonates. Often, fever is the only sign, although the majority of neonates with fever have minor illnesses (96 to 97 percent). The few that are seriously ill can be easily missed. For this reason, any fever in a neonate requires extensive evaluation.

The approach to this age group should include several factors. First, the child should always be kept warm. Observe skin color, tone, and respiratory activity. The absence of tears when crying may indicate dehydration. The lungs should be auscultated early during the exam, while the infant is quiet. You might find it helpful to have the child suck on a pacifier during the examination. Allowing the infant to remain in a parent's or caregiver's lap may help keep the child calm. Obviously, the history must be obtained from the parents or caregivers. However, it is also important to observe the child.

Infants (1 to 5 Months) pp. 74–75

Infants should have doubled their birth weight by 5 to 6 months of age. They should be able to follow the movements of others with their eyes. Muscle control develops in a cephalocaudal progression. This means, literally, that development of muscular control begins at the head (*cephalo*) and moves toward the tail (*caudal*). Muscular control also spreads from the trunk toward the extremities during this period. The infant's personality at this stage still centers closely on the parents or caregivers. The history must be obtained from these individuals, with close attention to possible illnesses and accidents, including sudden infant death syndrome (SIDS), vomiting, dehydration, meningitis, child abuse, and household accidents.

Concentrate on keeping these patients warm and comfortable. Allow the infant to remain in the parent's or caregiver's lap. A pacifier or bottle can be used to help keep the baby quiet during the examination.

Infants (6 to 12 Months) p. 75

Infants in this age group may stand or even walk with assistance. They are quite active and enjoy exploring the world with their mouths. In this stage of development, the risk of foreign body airway

©2013 Pearson Education, Inc.
Paramedic Care: Principles & Practice, Vol. 6, 4th Ed.

obstruction (FBAO) becomes a serious concern. Infants 6 months and older have more fully formed personalities and express themselves more readily. They have considerable anxiety toward strangers. They do not like lying on their backs. Children in this age group tend to cling to the mother, although the father "will do" in many cases. Common illnesses and accidents include febrile seizures, vomiting, diarrhea, dehydration, bronchiolitis, car crashes, croup, child abuse, poisonings, falls, airway obstructions, and meningitis.

These children should be examined while sitting in the lap of the parent or caregiver. The exam should progress in a toe-to-head order, since because starting at the face may upset the child. If time and conditions permit, allow the child to become familiar with you before beginning the examination.

Toddlers (1 to 3 Years) p. 75
Great strides occur in gross motor development during this stage. Children tend to run underneath or stand on almost everything. They seem to always be on the move. As they grow older, toddlers become braver and more curious or stubborn. They begin to stray away from the parents or caregivers more frequently. These remain the only people who can comfort them quickly, however, and most children will cling to a parent or caregiver if frightened. At ages 1 to 3 years, language development begins. Often children can understand better than they can speak. Therefore, the majority of the medical history will still come from the parents or caregivers. Remember, however, that you can ask toddlers simple and specific questions.

Accidents of all types are the leading cause of injury deaths in pediatric patients ages 1 to 15 years. Common accidents in this age group include motor vehicle collisions, homicides, burn injuries, drownings, and pedestrian collisions. Common illnesses and injuries in the toddler age group include vomiting, diarrhea, febrile seizures, poisonings, falls, child abuse, croup, and meningitis. Keep in mind that FBAO is still a high risk for toddlers.

Be cautious when treating toddlers. Approach toddlers slowly and try to gain their confidence. Conduct the exam in a toe-to-head order. The child may be difficult to examine and may resist being touched. Speak quietly and use only simple words. Avoid asking questions that allow the child to say "no." If the situation permits, allow toddlers to hold transitional objects such as a favorite blanket or toy. Be sure to tell the child if something will hurt. If at all possible, avoid procedures on the dominant arm/hand, which the child will try to pull away.

Preschoolers (3 to 5 Years) p. 75
Children in this age group show a tremendous increase in fine and gross motor development. Language skills increase greatly. Children in this age group know how to talk. However, if frightened, they often refuse to speak, especially to strangers. They often have vivid imaginations and may see monsters as part of their world. Preschoolers may have tempers and will express them. During this stage of development, children fear mutilation and may feel threatened by treatment. Avoid frightening or misleading comments. Preschoolers often run to a particular parent or caregiver, depending on the occasion. They stick up for the people they love and are openly affectionate. They still seek support and comfort from within the home.

When evaluating children in this age group, question the child first, keeping in mind that imagination may interfere with the facts. The child often has a distorted sense of time; thus, you must rely on the parents or caregivers to fill in the gaps. Common illnesses, accidents, and injuries in this age group include croup, asthma, poisonings, auto collisions, burns, child abuse, ingestion of foreign bodies, drownings, epiglottitis, febrile seizures, and meningitis.

Treatment of preschoolers requires tact. Avoid baby talk. If time and situation permit, give the child health care choices. Often the use of a doll or stuffed animal will assist in the examination. Allow the child to hold a piece of equipment, such as a stethoscope, and to use it. Let the child sit on your lap. Start the examination with the chest and evaluate the head last. Avoid misleading comments. Do not trick or lie to the child and always explain what you are going to do.

School-Age Children (6 to 12 Years) p. 76
Children in this age group are active and carefree. Growth spurts sometimes lead to clumsiness. The personality continues to develop. School-age children are protective and proud of their parents or caregivers and seek their attention. They value peers, but also need home support.

When examining school-age children, give them the responsibility of providing the history. However, remember that children may be reluctant to provide information if they sustained an injury while doing something forbidden. The parents or caregivers can fill in the pertinent details. When assessing children in this age group, it is important to respect their modesty. Be honest and tell the child what is wrong. A small toy may help to calm the child. Common illnesses and injuries for this age group include drownings, auto collisions, bicycle accidents, falls, fractures, sports injuries, child abuse, and burns.

Adolescents (13 to 18 Years) p. 76

Adolescence covers the period from the end of childhood to the start of adulthood (age 18). It begins with puberty, roughly age 13 for male children and age 11 for female children. (For this reason, adolescence is often defined as including ages 11 to 18, rather than 13 to 18.) Puberty is highly child specific and can begin at various ages. A female child, for example, may experience her first menstrual period as early as age 7 or 8. Adolescents vary significantly in their development. Those over age 15 are physically nearer to adults in terms of their vital signs, but emotionally they may still be children. They worry about their physical image more than any other pediatric age group. You should tactfully address their stated concerns about body integrity or disfigurement. The slightest possibility of a lasting scar may be a tremendous issue to the adolescent patient.

Although patients in this age group are not yet legally adults, most consider themselves to be grown up. They take offense at the use of the word "child." They have a strong desire to be liked by their peers and to be included. Relationships with parents and caregivers may at times be strained as the adolescent demands greater independence. They value the opinions of other adolescents, especially members of the opposite sex. Generally, these patients make good historians. Do not be surprised, however, if their perception of events differs from that of their parents or caregivers.

Common illnesses and injuries in this age group include mononucleosis, asthma, auto collisions, sports injuries, drug and alcohol problems, suicide gestures, and sexual abuse. Remember that pregnancy is also possible in female adolescents. When assessing teenagers, remember that vital signs will approach those of adults. In gathering a history, be factual and address the patient's questions. It may be wise to interview the patient away from the parents or caregivers. Listen to what the teenager is saying, as well as what he is not saying. If you suspect substance abuse or endangerment of the patient or others, approach the subject with tact and compassion. If you must perform a detailed physical exam, respect the teenager's sense of privacy. If the patient exhibits modesty or bodily shame, have a paramedic of the same sex as the teenager conduct the examination, if possible. Regardless of the situation, provide psychological support and reassurance.

5. **Consider the psychosocial needs of the parents or caregivers of a pediatric patient.** p. 74

Care for the pediatric patient also involves the family members or caregivers responsible for the child. They will demand information, express fears, and, ultimately, give or refuse consent for treatment and/or transport. Interaction with pediatric patients and related adults continues throughout assessment and management. Pay attention to the way in which parents or caregivers interact with the child. Are the interactions appropriate to the emergency? Are family members concerned? Are they angry? Are they overly emotional or entirely indifferent?

6. **Use a process of clinical reasoning to guide and interpret the patient assessment and management process for pediatric patients.** p. 80

Priorities in the management of the pediatric patient, as with all patients, are established on a threat-to-life basis. If life-threatening problems are not present, you will complete each of the general steps discussed in the following sections. Whenever possible, involve the parent or caregiver in efforts to calm or comfort the child. Depending on the situation, you may decide to allow the parent or caregiver to remain with the child during treatment and transport.

From the time of dispatch, you will continually acquire information relative to the patient's condition. As with all patients, personal safety must be your first priority. In treating pediatric patients, follow the same guidelines in approaching the scene as you would with any other patient. Remember that infants and young children are at especially high risk of an infectious process.

©2013 Pearson Education, Inc.

Paramedic Care: Principles & Practice, Vol. 6, 4th Ed.

7. **Adapt the scene size-up, primary assessment, patient history, secondary assessment, and use of monitoring technology to meet the needs of pediatric patients.**   pp. 80–89

On arrival, conduct a quick scene size-up. Dispatch information received en route, as well as your own observations, can provide critical indicators of scene safety. As you survey the scene, look for clues to the mechanism of injury (MOI) or the nature of the illness (NOI). These clues will help guide your assessment and determine appropriate interventions. Remain alert for evidence of child abuse, particularly in cases in which the injury and history do not coincide. As already mentioned, pay attention to the way parents or caregivers respond to the child and the way the child responds to them. Pace your approach to give the child time to adjust to your presence. Speak in a soft voice, using simple words. As soon as you reach the child, position yourself at eye level with the patient and make every effort to win his trust. If the child bonds more readily with one member of the team than another, allow that person to remain with the child and, if possible, allow that person to conduct most of the secondary assessment.

The patient's condition determines the course of your primary assessment. An active and alert child will allow for a more comfortable approach, with more time spent on communication with the child and appropriate adults. A critically ill or injured child, however, may require quick intervention and rapid transport. Your choice of action depends on your general impression of the patient. The major points in forming your general impression are outlined in an assessment tool called the pediatric assessment triangle. The triangle's three components are: appearance (mental status and muscle tone), breathing (respiratory rate and effort), and circulation (skin signs and color and capillary refill).

Employ the AVPU method to evaluate the pediatric patient's level of consciousness. Adjust the techniques for the child's age. Assess the airway for patency and maintainability. If at any point the patient shows little or no movement of air, intervene immediately. Keep this fact in mind: Airway and respiratory problems are the most common cause of cardiac arrest in infants and young children. Assess breathing. Look at the patient's chest and abdomen for movement. Listen for breath sounds. Feel for air movement at the patient's mouth. Your goal is to identify any evidence of compromised breathing. Evaluation of breathing includes assessment of the following conditions: respiratory rate, respiratory effort, and color. In general, evaluate the following conditions when assessing circulation during the primary assessment: heart rate, peripheral circulation, and end-organ perfusion. Remember that evaluation of mental status and ABCs during the primary assessment is rapid and not detailed because it is aimed at discovering and correcting immediate life threats. Based on your primary assessment, you will assign the patient as an urgent or nonurgent priority for transport.

After you have prioritized patient care at the end of the primary assessment, you will perform the secondary assessment, including a history and a physical exam. If the patient has a medical illness, the history will precede the physical exam. If the patient is suffering from trauma, the physical exam will take precedence.

To obtain a history for a pediatric patient, you will probably need to involve a family member or caregiver. Remember, however, that school-age children and adolescents like to take part in their own care. As previously mentioned, you can elicit valuable information from even very young patients. As a general precaution, question older adolescent patients in private, especially about issues such as sexual activity, pregnancy, or illicit drug and alcohol use. As with any patient, you will use the history to uncover additional pertinent injuries or medical conditions. The history should center on the chief complaint and past medical history. The past medical history identifies chronic illnesses, use of medications, and allergies. Be sure to inquire whether the infant or child is currently under a doctor's care. If so, obtain the name of the physician and present it at the receiving hospital.

Carry out the physical exam after all life-threatening conditions have been identified and addressed. If there is a significant mechanism of injury or if the patient is unresponsive, perform a complete rapid trauma assessment or rapid medical assessment. Use the toe-to-head approach with the younger child (or begin with the chest and examine the head last) and the head-to-toe approach in the older child.

In cases of trauma, you may need to apply the Glasgow Coma Scale (GCS), a scoring system for monitoring the neurological status of patients with possible head injuries. The GCS assigns scores based on verbal responses, motor functions, and eye movements. In using the GCS with pediatric patients, you will have to make certain modifications. After you score the GCS for the patient, prioritize the patient according to severity. Guidelines are as follows: mild (GCS 13 to 15), moderate (GCS 9 to 12), and severe (GCS less than or equal to 8).

Remember that poorly taken vital signs are of less value than no vital signs at all. Take vital signs with the patient in as close to a resting state as possible. Obtain blood pressure with an appropriate-sized cuff. Feel for peripheral, brachial, or femoral pulses. It is generally not possible to weigh the child. However, if medications are required, make a good estimate of the child's weight. Observe the child's respiratory rate before beginning the examination. Measure temperature early in the patient encounter and repeat toward the end. Continue to observe the child for level of consciousness.

To promote the goal of early recognition of cardiopulmonary arrest, every seriously ill or injured child should receive continuous pulse oximetry. This will provide you with essential information regarding the patient's heart rate and peripheral O_2 saturation. The goal is to maintain an SpO_2 of 94 percent or greater. Capnography, also called end-tidal carbon dioxide monitoring ($PETCO_2$), is useful in pediatrics. It provides essential information about ventilation and can also provide diagnostic information. If the $PETCO_2$ is consistently greater than 10 to 15 mmHg, focus efforts on improving chest compressions and make sure that the patient does not receive excessive ventilation (hyperventilation). An electrocardiogram (ECG) and automated blood pressure/pulse monitor should also be considered. However, these devices may frighten the child. Before applying any monitoring device, explain what you are going to do. Demonstrate the display or lights. If the monitoring device makes noise, allow the child to hear the noise before you apply it. Reassure the child that the device will not hurt him.

Because a pediatric patient's condition can rapidly change for the better or the worse, it is necessary to repeat relevant portions of the assessment. You should continually monitor the patient's respiratory effort, skin color, mental status, temperature, and pulse oximetry. Retake vital signs and compare them with baseline vitals. In general, reassess stable patients every 15 minutes, critical patients every 5 minutes.

8. **Recognize specific problems in pediatric patients, including infection, respiratory emergencies, hypoperfusion, cardiac emergencies, neurologic emergencies, gastrointestinal problems, diabetic emergencies, poisoning and toxicologic emergencies, trauma, drowning, and burns.**

Infection

p. 106

Childhood is a time of frequent illnesses because of the relative immaturity of the pediatric immune system. Infectious diseases may be caused by the infection or infestation of the body by an infectious agent such as a virus, bacterium, fungus, or parasite. Most infections are minor and self-limiting. Several infections, however, can be life threatening. These include meningitis, pneumonia, and septicemia, a systemic infection (usually bacterial) in the bloodstream. The impact of an infection on physiological processes depends on the type of infectious agent and the extent of the infection.

Respiratory Emergencies

pp. 106–112

Respiratory emergencies constitute the most common reason EMS is summoned to care for a pediatric patient. The mildest form of respiratory impairment is classified as respiratory distress. Respiratory failure occurs when the respiratory system is not able to meet the demands of the body for oxygen intake and for carbon dioxide removal. The end result of respiratory impairment, if untreated, is respiratory arrest. The cessation of breathing typically follows a period of bradypnea and agonal respirations.

Croup. Croup, medically referred to as laryngotracheobronchitis, is a viral infection of the upper airway. It most commonly occurs in children 6 months to 4 years of age and is prevalent in the fall and winter. Croup causes an inflammation of the upper respiratory tract involving the subglottic region. The infection leads to edema beneath the glottis and larynx, thus narrowing the lumen of the airway. Severe cases of croup can lead to complete airway obstruction. Another form of croup, called spasmodic croup, occurs mostly in the middle of the night without any prior upper respiratory infection.

Epiglottitis. Epiglottitis is an acute infection and inflammation of the epiglottis and is potentially life threatening. Epiglottitis, unlike croup, is caused by a bacterial infection, usually *Haemophilus influenzae* type B. As a result of the availability of the *H. influenzae* vaccination, epiglottitis has become an uncommon occurrence. When it does occur, it tends to strike children aged 3 to 7 years old.

©2013 Pearson Education, Inc.

Paramedic Care: Principles & Practice, Vol. 6, 4th Ed.

Bacterial Tracheitis. Bacterial tracheitis is a bacterial infection of the airway in the subglottic region. Although the condition is very uncommon, it is most likely to appear following episodes of viral croup. It afflicts mainly infants and toddlers 1 to 5 years of age.

Foreign Body Aspiration. Children, especially 1- to 4-year-olds, like to put objects into their mouths. As a result, these children are at increased risk of aspirating foreign bodies, especially when they run or fall. In fact, foreign body aspiration is the number one cause of in-home accidental deaths in children under 6 years of age. Common foods associated with aspiration and airway obstruction in children include hard candy, nuts, seeds, hot dogs, sausages, and grapes. Nonfood items include coins, balloons, and other small objects.

Asthma. Asthma is a chronic inflammatory disorder of the airways, characterized by bronchospasm and excessive mucous production. In susceptible children, this inflammation causes widespread, but variable, airflow obstruction. In addition to airflow obstruction, the airways become hyperresponsive. Within minutes of exposure to the trigger, a two-phase reaction occurs. The first phase of the reaction is characterized by the release of chemical mediators such as histamine. These cause bronchoconstriction and bronchial edema that effectively decrease expiratory airflow, causing the classic "asthma attack." The second phase is characterized by inflammation of the bronchioles as cells of the immune system invade the respiratory tract. This causes additional edema and further decreases expiratory airflow. Status asthmaticus is defined as a severe, prolonged asthma attack that cannot be broken by aggressive pharmacologic management. This is a serious medical emergency. Prompt recognition, treatment, and transport are required.

Bronchiolitis. Bronchiolitis is a respiratory infection of the medium-sized airways that occurs in early childhood. It should not be confused with bronchitis, which is an infection of the larger bronchi. Bronchiolitis is caused by a viral infection, most commonly respiratory syncytial virus (RSV) that affects the lining of the bronchioles. Bronchiolitis is characterized by prominent expiratory wheezing and clinically resembles asthma. It most commonly occurs in winter in children less than 2 years of age.

Pneumonia. Pneumonia is an infection of the lower airway and lungs. Either a bacterium or a virus may cause it. Pneumonia can occur at any age, but in pediatric patients, it most commonly appears in infants, toddlers, and preschoolers aged 1 to 5 years. Most cases of pneumonia in children are viral and self-limited. As children get older, they can contract bacterial pneumonias like adults do.

Foreign Body Lower Airway Obstruction. A foreign body can enter the lower airway if it is too small to lodge in the upper airway. Depending on positioning, the foreign body can act as a one-way valve and either trap air in distal lung tissues or prevent aeration of distal lung tissues, causing a ventilation/perfusion mismatch.

Hypoperfusion   pp. 112–114

Hypovolemic Shock. Hypovolemic shock results from loss of intravascular fluids. In pediatric patients, the most common causes include severe dehydration from vomiting and/or diarrhea and blood loss, usually as a result of trauma. Trauma may include blood loss into a body cavity (particularly the abdomen) or frank external hemorrhage. Children are also at risk of fluid loss as a result of burns, the second leading cause of pediatric deaths in the United States.

Septic Shock. This condition is caused by sepsis, an infection of the bloodstream by some pathogen, usually bacterial. Sepsis commonly occurs as a complication of an infection at some other site, such as pneumonia, an ear infection, or a urinary tract infection.

Anaphylactic Shock. Anaphylactic shock results from exposure to an antigen to which the patient has been previously exposed. Milder cases may simply result in an allergic reaction. More severe reactions can impair tissue perfusion. This primarily occurs as a result of the release of histamine and other similar chemicals. Histamine causes peripheral vasodilation and leakage of fluid from the intravascular space into the interstitial space.

Neurogenic Shock. Neurogenic shock is due to sudden peripheral vasodilation resulting from interruption of nervous control of the peripheral vascular system. The most common cause is injury to the spinal cord. Cardiac output and intravascular fluid volume are usually adequate.

Cardiogenic Shock. Cardiogenic shock results from inadequate cardiac output. In children, cardiogenic shock usually results from a secondary cause such as near drowning or a toxic ingestion. Children, unlike adults, rarely have primary cardiac disease. The exceptions are congenital heart disease and cardiomyopathy. Congenital heart disease is an abnormality or defect in the heart that is present at birth. Cardiomyopathy is a disease or dysfunction of the cardiac muscle.

Cardiac Emergencies
pp. 114–116

Supraventricular Tachycardia. True supraventricular tachycardia (SVT) is a narrow-complex tachycardia (QRS ≤ 0.09 second) with a heart rate typically of 220 beats per minute or greater. Supraventricular tachycardia is usually caused by a problem in the cardiac conductive system. Rarely, it can be the result of a secondary cause such as drug ingestion. It is occasionally seen in infants with no prior history. The cause is uncertain but may be due to immaturity of the cardiac conductive system. Rapid heart rates often do not allow time for adequate cardiac filling, eventually causing congestive heart failure and cardiogenic shock.

Ventricular Tachycardia with a Pulse. Ventricular tachycardia (wide-complex tachycardia) and ventricular fibrillation are exceedingly rare in children. They are occasionally seen following near-drowning or following a prolonged resuscitation attempt. Unlike adults, in whom ventricular tachyarrhythmias result from primary heart disease, ventricular tachyarrhythmias in children are almost always due to a secondary cause. The exception is structural, congenital heart disease.

Bradyarrhythmias. Bradyarrhythmias are the most common type of pediatric arrhythmia. They most frequently result from hypoxia. Although rare, they can also result from vagal stimulation from such causes as marked gastric distention.

Asystole. Asystole is the absence of a rhythm and may be the initial rhythm seen in cardiopulmonary arrest. (Remember that children rarely develop ventricular fibrillation, which is often the precursor to arrest in adults.) Bradycardias can degenerate to asystole if appropriate intervention is not provided. The mortality rate associated with asystole in children is very high.

Ventricular Fibrillation/Pulseless Ventricular Tachycardia. Ventricular fibrillation and pulseless ventricular tachycardia are functionally the same rhythm. They are exceedingly rare in children. Causes include electrocution and drug overdoses. The mortality rate is very high.

Pulseless Electrical Activity. Pulseless electrical activity (PEA) is the presence of a cardiac rhythm without an associated pulse. This is due to noncardiogenic causes such as hypoxia, pericardial tamponade, tension pneumothorax, trauma, acidosis, hypothermia, and hypoglycemia.

Neurologic Emergencies
pp. 116–117

Seizures. Seizures result from an abnormal discharge of neurons in the brain. Although the etiology for seizures is often unknown, several risk factors have been identified, including: fever, hypoxia, infections, idiopathic epilepsy (unknown origin), electrolyte disturbances, head trauma, hypoglycemia, toxic ingestions or exposure, tumor, and central nervous system (CNS) malformations.

Seizures in pediatric patients may be either partial or generalized. Simple partial seizures, sometimes called focal motor seizures, involve sudden jerking of a particular part of the body, such as an arm or a leg. Other characteristics include lip smacking, eye blinking, staring, confusion, and lethargy. There is usually no loss of consciousness. Generalized seizures involve sudden jerking of both sides of the body, followed by tenseness and relaxation of the body. In a generalized seizure, patients typically experience a loss of consciousness.

Keep in mind that children can have status epilepticus, a series of one or more generalized seizures, without any intervening periods of consciousness. Status epilepticus is a serious medical emergency because it involves a prolonged period of apnea, which in turn can cause hypoxia of vital brain tissues. Most of the pediatric seizures that you will probably encounter are febrile seizures. Febrile seizures are those seizures that occur as a result of a sudden increase in body temperature. They occur most commonly between the ages of 6 months and 6 years. Often, the parents or caregivers will report the recent onset of fever or cold symptoms. The diagnosis of febrile seizure should not be made in the field. All

©2013 Pearson Education, Inc.
Paramedic Care: Principles & Practice, Vol. 6, 4th Ed.

pediatric patients suffering a seizure must be transported to the hospital so that other etiologies can be excluded.

Meningitis. Meningitis is an infection of the meninges, the lining of the brain and spinal cord. Meningitis can result from both bacteria and viruses. Viral meningitis is frequently called aseptic meningitis, because an organism cannot be routinely cultured from cerebrospinal fluid (CSF). Aseptic meningitis is generally less severe than bacterial meningitis and is self-limiting. Bacterial meningitis most commonly results from *Streptococcus pneumoniae*, *Haemophilus influenzae*, and *Neisseria meningitides*. These infections can be rapidly fatal if they are not promptly recognized and treated appropriately.

Gastrointestinal Problems   pp. 117–118

Nausea and Vomiting. Nausea and vomiting are not diseases themselves, but are symptoms of other disease processes. Virtually any medical problem can cause these conditions in an infant or child. The most common causes include fever, ear infections, and respiratory infections. In addition, many viruses and certain bacteria can infect the gastrointestinal system. These infections, collectively known as gastroenteritis, readily cause vomiting, diarrhea, or both. The biggest risks associated with nausea and vomiting in children are dehydration and electrolyte abnormalities. Infants and toddlers can quickly become dehydrated from bouts of vomiting. If diarrhea or fever is also present, fluid loss is further accelerated, worsening the situation. Dehydration is more difficult to detect in infants and toddlers than in older children.

Diarrhea. Diarrhea is a common occurrence in childhood. Often, what parents call diarrhea is actually loose bowel movements. Generally, 10 or more stools per day is considered diarrhea. As with nausea and vomiting, the main concern associated with diarrhea is dehydration. Most diarrhea is caused by viral infections of the gastrointestinal system or arises secondary to infections elsewhere in the body. However, certain bacterial infections can cause significant, even life-threatening, diarrhea.

Diabetic Emergencies   pp. 118–119

Hypoglycemia. Hypoglycemia is an abnormally low concentration of sugar (glucose) in the blood. It is a true medical emergency that must be treated immediately. Without treatment, a low blood sugar may progress to unconsciousness and convulsions. In the prehospital setting, hypoglycemia in pediatric patients usually occurs in newborn infants and children with type 1 diabetes. Diabetic children increase their risk of hypoglycemia through overly strenuous exercise, too much insulin, and dehydration from illness. Nondiabetic children can develop hypoglycemia from physical activity, diet changes, illness, and growth.

Hyperglycemia. Hyperglycemia is an abnormally high concentration of blood sugar. For patients with type 1 diabetes, hyperglycemia may lead to dehydration and diabetic ketoacidosis, a very serious medical emergency. Left untreated, the condition will deteriorate to coma. Hyperglycemia and diabetic ketoacidosis are the most common findings in new-onset diabetics. In the prehospital setting, pediatric hyperglycemia is commonly associated with type 1 diabetes. Causes include eating too much food relative to injected insulin; missing an insulin injection; defective insulin pump, blockage of tubing, or disconnection of insulin pump infusion set; and illness or stress. Hyperglycemia can occur with other severe illnesses and not necessarily mean that the child is developing diabetes mellitus.

Poisoning and Toxicologic Emergencies   pp. 119–121
Pediatric patients account for the majority of poisonings treated by EMS. Most poisonings result from accidental ingestion of a toxic substance, usually by a young child. Toddlers and preschoolers like to taste things, especially colorful objects and substances that look like food or beverages.

Poisonings are the leading cause of preventable death in children under age 5. The best way to prevent pediatric poisonings is by helping the families in your communities learn how to "poison-proof" their homes.

Trauma   pp. 121–126
Trauma is the number one cause of death in infants and children. Most pediatric injuries result from blunt trauma. If you serve in an urban area, you can expect to see a higher incidence of penetrating

trauma, mostly intentional and mostly from gunfire or knife wounds. Significant incidences of penetrating trauma are also seen outside the cities, mostly unintentional, from hunting accidents and agricultural accidents.

Traumatic Brain Injury. Children, because of the relatively large size of their heads and weak neck muscles, are at increased risk for traumatic brain injury. These injuries can be devastating and are often fatal. Early recognition and aggressive management can reduce both morbidity and mortality. Pediatric head injuries can be classified as follows: mild (Glascow coma score [GCS] 13–15), moderate (GSC 9–12), and severe (GSC less than or equal to 8).

Head, Face, and Neck. The majority of children who sustain multiple traumas will suffer associated head and/or neck injuries. Injuries to the head are the most common cause of death in pediatric trauma victims. School-age children tend to sustain head injuries from bicycle collisions, falls from trees, or car–pedestrian collisions. Older children most commonly suffer head injuries from sporting events. Heads injuries in all age groups may result from abuse. The most common facial injuries are lacerations secondary to falls. Young children are very clumsy when they first start walking. A fall onto a sharp object, such as the corner of a coffee table, can result in a laceration. Older children sustain dental injuries in falls from bicycles, skateboard accidents, fights, and sports activities. Spinal injuries in children are not as common as in adults. A child's proportionately larger and heavier head makes the cervical spine vulnerable to injury. Any time a child sustains a severe head injury, always assume that a neck injury may also be present.

Injuries to the Chest. Chest injuries are the second most common cause of pediatric trauma deaths. Pneumothorax and hemothorax can occur in the pediatric patient, especially if the mechanism of injury was a motor vehicle collision. Tension pneumothorax can also occur in children. Pediatric patients poorly tolerate the condition and a needle thoracostomy may be a lifesaving measure.

Injuries to the Abdomen. Significant blunt trauma to the abdomen can result in injury to the spleen or liver. In fact, the spleen is the most commonly injured organ in children.

Extremities. Extremity injuries in children are typically limited to fractures and lacerations. Children rarely sustain amputations and other serious extremity injuries. An exception is farm children, who may become entangled in agricultural equipment. The most common injuries are fractures, usually resulting from falls. Because children have more flexible bones than adults, they tend to have incomplete fractures, such as bend fractures, buckle fractures, and greenstick fractures. In younger children, the bone growth plates have not yet closed. Some types of growth plate fractures can lead to permanent disability if not managed correctly. Whenever indicated, perform splinting in order to decrease pain and prevent further injury and/or blood loss.

Drownings and Near Drownings   pp. 122–123

Drowning is the third leading cause of death in children between birth and 4 years of age, with approximately 2,000 deaths occurring in the United States annually. The term *drowning* is used to describe deaths that occur within 24 hours of the incident. Near-drowning refers to injuries in which the child did not die or where the death occurred more than 24 hours after the injury. Many children who do not die from drowning suffer severe and irreversible brain injuries as a result of anoxia. Approximately 20 percent to 25 percent of near-drowning survivors exhibit severe neurologic deficits. The outcomes are better when the water is cold, because the body's protective mechanisms protect against brain injury.

Burns   pp. 123; 126–127

Burns are the second leading cause of death in children. They are the leading cause of accidental death in the home for children under 14. Burns may be chemical, thermal, or electrical. The most common type of burn injury encountered by EMS personnel is scalding. Children can scald themselves by pulling hot liquids off tables or stoves. In cases of abuse, they can be scalded by immersion in hot water.

©2013 Pearson Education, Inc.
Paramedic Care: Principles & Practice, Vol. 6, 4th Ed.

9. **Relate the pathophysiology of specific pediatric problems to the priorities of patient assessment and management.**

Infection
p. 106

Signs and symptoms of infection may vary, depending on the type of infection and the time since exposure. Any of the following conditions may indicate the presence of an infection: fever, chills, tachycardia, cough, sore throat, nasal congestion, malaise, tachypnea, cool or clammy skin, petechiae, respiratory distress, poor appetite, vomiting, diarrhea, dehydration, hypoperfusion (especially with septicemia), purpura (purple blotches resulting from hemorrhages into the skin that do not disappear under pressure), seizures, severe headache, irritability, stiff neck, or bulging fontanelle (infants).

The management of infections depends on the body system or systems affected. As a general rule, you should adhere to these guidelines when treating an infectious illness: take Standard Precautions; become familiar with the common pediatric infections encountered in your area; and, if possible, try to determine which, if any, pediatric infections you have not been exposed to or vaccinated for.

Respiratory Emergencies
pp. 106–112

The signs and symptoms of respiratory distress include normal mental status deteriorating to irritability or anxiety, tachypnea, retractions, nasal flaring (in infants), poor muscle tone, tachycardia, head bobbing, grunting, and cyanosis or hypoxia that improves with supplemental oxygen. If not corrected immediately, respiratory distress will lead to respiratory failure.

The signs and symptoms of respiratory failure include irritability or anxiety deteriorating to lethargy, marked tachypnea later deteriorating to bradypnea, marked retractions later deteriorating to agonal respirations, poor muscle tone, marked tachycardia later deteriorating to bradycardia, central cyanosis, and hypoxia. Respiratory failure is a very ominous sign. If immediate intervention is not provided, the child will deteriorate to full respiratory arrest.

Signs and symptoms of respiratory arrest include unresponsiveness deteriorating to coma, bradypnea deteriorating to apnea, absent chest wall motion, bradycardia deteriorating to asystole, and profound cyanosis. Respiratory arrest will quickly deteriorate to full cardiopulmonary arrest if appropriate interventions are not made. The child's chances of survival markedly decrease when cardiopulmonary arrest occurs.

Croup. The history for croup is fairly classic. Often, the child will have a mild cold or other infection and be doing fairly well until evening. After dark, however, a harsh, barking, or brassy cough develops. The attack may subside in a few hours but can persist for several nights. The physical exam will often reveal inspiratory stridor. There may be associated nasal flaring, tracheal tugging, or retraction.

Management of croup consists of appropriate airway maintenance. Place the child in a position of comfort and administer cool mist air or oxygen by face mask or the blow-by method. If the attack is severe, the physician may order the administration of racemic epinephrine or albuterol.

Epiglottitis. Epiglottitis presents similarly to croup. Often the child will go to bed feeling relatively well, usually with what parents or caregivers consider to be a mild infection of the respiratory tract. Later, the child awakens with a high temperature and a brassy cough. The progression of symptoms can be dramatic. There is often pain upon swallowing, sore throat, high fever, shallow breathing, dyspnea, inspiratory stridor, and drooling. On physical examination, the child will appear acutely ill and agitated. In epiglottitis, the epiglottis is cherry red and swollen. As airway obstruction develops, the child will exhibit retractions, nasal flaring, and pulmonary hyperexpansion. As the epiglottis swells, he may not be able to swallow his saliva and will begin to drool. Often the child will want to remain seated. Patients will often assume the "tripod position" to help maximize their airway.

Management of epiglottitis consists of appropriate airway maintenance and oxygen administration by face mask or the blow-by technique. Ideally, the oxygen should be humidified to minimize drying of the epiglottis and airway. To reduce the child's anxiety, you might ask the parent or caregiver to administer the oxygen. If the airway becomes obstructed, two-rescuer ventilation with a bag-valve mask (BVM) is almost always effective. Remember, however, that intubation is contraindicated unless complete obstruction has occurred. Pediatric patients with epiglottitis require immediate transport. Handle the child gently, as stress could lead to total airway obstruction from spasms of the larynx and swelling tissues. Avoid IV sticks, do not take a blood pressure, and do not attempt to look into the mouth. During transport, reassure and comfort the child. Constantly monitor the child, and notify the hospital of any changes in status. Remember, if the patient is maintaining his airway, do not put anything in the child's mouth, including a thermometer. At all times, consider epiglottitis a critical condition.

Bacterial Tracheitis. In assessing bacterial tracheitis, parents or caregivers will typically report that the child has experienced an episode of croup in the preceding few days. They will also indicate the presence of a high-grade fever accompanied by coughing up of pus and/or mucus. The patient may exhibit a hoarse voice and, if able to talk, the child may complain of a sore throat. A physical examination may reveal inspiratory or expiratory stridor. As with all respiratory emergencies, the child must be carefully monitored, as respiratory failure or arrest may be an end result.

Carefully manage airway and breathing, providing oxygenation by face mask or the blow-by technique. Keep in mind that ventilations may require high pressure in order to adequately ventilate the patient. This may require depressing the pop-off valve of the pediatric BVM device, if the valve is present. Consider intubation only in cases of complete airway obstruction. Transport guidelines are similar to those for cases of epiglottitis.

Foreign Body Aspiration. The child with a suspected aspirated foreign body may present in one of two ways. If the obstruction is complete, the child will have minimal or no air movement. If the obstruction is partial, the child may exhibit inspiratory stridor, a muffled or hoarse voice, drooling, pain in the throat, retractions, and cyanosis.

If the obstruction is partial, make the child as comfortable as possible and administer humidified oxygen. If the child is old enough, place him in a sitting position. Do not attempt to look in the mouth. Transport the child to a hospital, where the foreign body can be removed by hospital personnel in a controlled environment.

If the obstruction is complete, clear the airway with accepted basic life-support (BLS) techniques. Sweep visible obstructions with your gloved finger. Do not perform blind finger sweeps, because this can push a foreign body deeper into the airway. Following BLS foreign body removal procedures, attempt ventilation with a BVM. If unsuccessful, visualize the airway with a laryngoscope. If the foreign body is seen and readily accessible, try to remove it with Magill forceps. Intubate if possible. Continue BLS foreign body removal procedures. If the airway cannot be cleared by routine measures, consider needle cricothyrotomy per medical direction and only as a last resort. Transport following appropriate guidelines, avoiding further agitation of the child.

Asthma. In many cases, there is a prior history of asthma or reactive airway disease. On physical examination, the child is usually sitting up, leaning forward, and tachypneic. Often, there is an associated unproductive cough. Accessory respiratory muscle usage is usually evident. Wheezing may be heard. However, in a severe attack, the patient may not wheeze at all. This is an ominous finding. Some children will not wheeze, but will cough, often continuously. Generally there is associated tachycardia; this should be monitored, as virtually all medications used to treat asthma increase the heart rate. Pulse oximetry and capnography can help assess the severity of asthma and guide treatment. The primary therapeutic goals in the asthmatic patient are to correct hypoxia, reverse bronchospasm, and decrease inflammation. First, it is imperative that you establish an airway. Next, administer supplemental, humidified oxygen as necessary to correct hypoxia. Initial pharmacological therapy is the administration of an inhaled beta agonist.

The child suffering status asthmaticus will have a greatly distended chest from continued air trapping. Breath sounds, and often wheezing, may be absent. The patient is usually exhausted, severely acidotic, and often dehydrated. The management of status asthmaticus is basically the same as for asthma. However, you should recognize that respiratory arrest is imminent and remain prepared for endotracheal intubation. Transport should be immediate, with aggressive treatment continued en route.

Bronchiolitis. A history is necessary to distinguish bronchiolitis from asthma. Often, with bronchiolitis, there is a family history of asthma or allergies, although neither is yet present in the child. In addition, a low-grade fever often exists. A major distinguishing factor is age. Asthma rarely occurs before the age of 1 year, whereas bronchiolitis is more frequent in this age group. Your physical examination should be systematic. Pay particular attention to the presence of crackles or wheezes. In addition, note any evidence of infection or respiratory distress.

Prehospital management of suspected bronchiolitis is much the same as with asthma. Place the child in a semisitting position, if old enough, and administer humidified oxygen by mask or blow-by method. Ventilations should be supported as necessary. Equipment for intubation should be readily

©2013 Pearson Education, Inc.
Paramedic Care: Principles & Practice, Vol. 6, 4th Ed.

available. If respiratory distress is present, consider administration of a bronchodilator by small-volume nebulizer. The cardiac rhythm should be monitored constantly. Pulse oximetry, if available, should be used continuously.

Pneumonia. Persons with pneumonia often have a history of a respiratory infection, such as a severe cold or bronchitis. Signs and symptoms include a low-grade fever, decreased breath sounds, crackles, rhonchi, and pain in the chest area. Conduct a systematic assessment of a patient with suspected pneumonia, paying particular attention to evidence of respiratory distress.

Prehospital management of pneumonia is supportive. Place the patient in a position of comfort. Ensure a patent airway and administer supplemental oxygen via a nonrebreather device. If respiratory failure is present, support ventilations with a BVM device. If prolonged ventilation will be required, perform endotracheal intubation. Transport the patient in a position of comfort. Provide emotional and psychological support to the parents.

Foreign Body Lower Airway Obstruction. If the object is fairly large and aspirated, then respiratory distress may be present. There is often considerable, often intractable, coughing. The child will be anxious and may have diminished breath sounds in the part of the chest affected by the foreign body. There may be crackles or rhonchi, usually unilateral. In some cases, there may be unilateral wheezing where some air is getting past the object. Unilateral wheezing should be considered to be due to an aspirated foreign body until proven otherwise.

The management of an aspirated foreign body is supportive. Place the child in a position of comfort and avoid agitation. Provide supplemental oxygen. Transport the child to a facility that has the capability of performing pediatric fiber-optic bronchoscopy. The bronchoscope can be used to visualize the airway and remove any foreign objects detected.

Hypoperfusion
pp. 112–114

Hypovolemic Shock. Treatment of hypovolemic shock involves administration of supplemental oxygen and establishment of intravenous access. This should be followed by a 20-mL/kg bolus of lactated Ringer's or normal saline. Following the bolus, the child should be reassessed. If signs and symptoms of compensated shock still exist, then administer a second bolus. Some children may require 80 to 100 mL/kg of fluid, depending on the volume of fluid lost.

Septic Shock. Signs and symptoms of septic shock include very ill appearance, altered mental status, tachycardia, capillary refill time greater than 2 seconds, hyperventilation leading to respiratory failure, cool and clammy skin, inability of child to recognize parents, and acidosis (elevated lactate) and/or increasing CO_2 levels. Supplemental oxygen should be administered and intravenous access obtained. Administer a 20-mL/kg bolus of lactated Ringer's or normal saline. Consider initiating pressor therapy with epinephrine or dopamine. Begin at the designated starting dose and gradually increase the dose until the blood pressure improves or there is evidence of improved end-organ perfusion. Definitive treatment includes antibiotics and other therapy. Transport should be rapid with care provided en route.

Anaphylactic Shock. Anaphylactic shock can be differentiated from a severe allergic reaction by the presence of signs and symptoms of impaired end-organ perfusion, including tachycardia, tachypnea, wheezing, urticaria (hives), anxiousness, edema, and hypotension. Treatment of anaphylactic shock includes supplemental oxygen administration and intravenous access. If the patient is exhibiting decompensated shock, administer epinephrine 1:10,000 intravenously and diphenhydramine (Benadryl) intravenously. Patients not exhibiting hypotension may be given an initial dose of epinephrine subcutaneously. If this does not rapidly improve the situation, then an intravenous dose of epinephrine should be considered. EMS systems with long transport times may be asked to administer an initial dose of a corticosteroid such as methylprednisolone (Solu-Medrol).

Neurogenic Shock. Treatment is directed at increasing peripheral vascular resistance. This is accomplished primarily through administration of a pressor agent such as dopamine. Care should also include stabilization of the injury and administration of supplemental oxygen (if the patient is hypoxic).

Cardiogenic Shock. The child with congenital heart disease may develop respiratory distress, congestive heart failure, or a "cyanotic spell." Cyanotic spells occur when oxygen demand exceeds that provided by the blood. They begin as irritability, inconsolable crying or altered mental status, and progressive cyanosis in conjunction with severe dyspnea. In severe and prolonged cases, seizures, coma, or cardiac arrest may result. Noncyanotic problems associated with congenital heart disease include respiratory distress, tachycardia, decreased end-organ perfusion, drowsiness, fatigue, and pallor. Treatment includes the standard primary assessment. Administer high-concentration oxygen. If necessary, provide ventilatory support. If the patient is having a cyanotic spell, place the child in the knee–chest position facing downward or, in an older child, have him squat. This will help increase the cardiac return. Apply the electrocardiogram (ECG) monitor, and start an intravenous line at a keep-open rate. Transport immediately.

The signs and symptoms of cardiomyopathy include early fatigue, crackles, jugular venous distention, engorgement of the liver, and peripheral edema. Later, as the disease progresses, the signs and symptoms of shock can develop. The prehospital treatment of cardiomyopathy is supportive. Supplemental oxygen should be administered via a nonrebreather mask. Fluids should be restricted. If possible, IV access should be obtained. Severe cases resulting in the development of severe dyspnea should be treated with furosemide and pressor agents (dobutamine, dopamine). The child should be transported to a facility capable of managing critically ill children. Most cases of cardiomyopathy are managed with medication. Definitive care in severe cases may include cardiac transplantation.

Cardiac Emergencies   pp. 114–116

Supraventricular Tachycardia. The signs and symptoms of supraventricular tachycardia include irritability, poor feeding, jugular venous distention, hepatomegaly (enlarged liver), and hypotension. The ECG will show a narrow complex (supraventricular) tachycardia with a rate greater than 220 beats per minute. Children can often tolerate the rapid rate well.

Prehospital treatment of supraventricular tachycardia depends on the clinical findings. Children who are tolerating the heart rate (normal blood pressure) and are stable should receive supplemental oxygen (if they are hypoxic) and transport. Vagal maneuvers may be attempted unless the patient is unstable. In older children, carotid sinus massage or Valsalva maneuvers are safe. Adenosine should be considered if the child is stable. If the child is exhibiting signs of decompensation (hypotension, mental status change, poor skin color), then synchronized cardioversion should be attempted at an initial energy dose of 0.5 to 1.0 joules per kilogram of body weight. This can be increased to 2 joules per kilogram if the initial shock is unsuccessful. Consider amiodarone 5 mg/kg IO/IV or procainamide 15 mg/kg IO/IV for a patient with supraventricular tachycardia (SVT) unresponsive to vagal maneuvers and adenosine and/or electric cardioversion. These medications must be administered slowly with all monitors in place. The child should be transported to the appropriate facility.

Ventricular Tachycardia with a Pulse. The signs and symptoms of ventricular tachycardia with a pulse include poor feeding, irritability, and a rapid, wide complex tachycardia. Children are unable to tolerate this arrhythmia very long. They soon develop signs of shock. The prehospital management includes supplemental oxygen and intravenous access. Stable patients who are not hypotensive should be transported. Unstable patients (hypotension) should be treated aggressively. Initially, amiodarone, procainamide, or lidocaine should be administered. However, ventricular tachycardia due to structural heart disease often does not respond to antiarrhythmic drugs. In stable children with wide-complex tachycardia, adenosine may be used to help distinguish supraventricular tachycardia from ventricular tachycardia (if the rhythm is regular and monomorphic). It may also convert supraventricular rhythms. Electrical cardioversion at 0.5 to 1.0 J/kg should be considered. This can be increased to 2 J/kg if needed. Pharmacological therapy should be considered (amiodarone or procainamide). In unstable children with wide-complex tachycardia, electrical cardioversion at 0.5 to 1.0 J/kg should be considered. This can be increased to 2 J/kg if needed.

Bradyarrhythmias. The signs and symptoms of bradycardia include a slow (usually < 60 beats per minute), narrow complex rhythm. The child may be lethargic, or exhibiting early signs of congestive heart failure. Stable children with bradyarrhyhmias should receive supportive care that addresses ventilation and oxygenation. If the heart rate falls below 60 beats per minute, they should be considered unstable. Unstable children (hypotension, altered mental status, signs of shock) should be ventilated with a BVM unit and 100 percent oxygen. If the heart rate does not increase readily, consider epinephrine intravenous (IV) or intraosseous (IO). Atropine may be used for suspected increased vagal tone of primary atrioventricular (AV) block. If pulseless arrest develops, perform chest compressions. If neces-

©2013 Pearson Education, Inc.
Paramedic Care: Principles & Practice, Vol. 6, 4th Ed.

sary, consider epinephrine or atropine down the endotracheal tube until IV or IO access can be obtained. Transport rapidly with care provided en route.

Asystole. The child with asystole is pulseless and apneic. The cardiac rhythm is a straight line that should be confirmed in two leads. Treatment is often futile. However, cardiopulmonary resuscitation (CPR) should be initiated, an IV or IO placed, and epinephrine administered every 3 to 5 minutes. The patient should be intubated and ventilated with 100 percent oxygen. Chest compressions should be continued. Emergency resuscitative drugs (epinephrine, atropine) should be administered through the endotracheal tube until intravenous access can be obtained.

Ventricular Fibrillation/Pulseless Ventricular Tachycardia. The child with ventricular fibrillation/ pulseless ventricular tachycardia will be pulseless and apneic. The ECG will exhibit a wide-complex tachycardia or fibrillation. The child should receive uninterrupted CPR for 2 minutes and IV/IO access should be obtained. After 2 minutes of CPR, the rhythm should be checked. If the patient is shockable, an initial shock of 2 J/kg should be provided and CPR resumed. Epinephrine should be administered every 3 to 5 minutes; an advanced airway should be placed and mechanical ventilation with 100 percent oxygen provided. If the patient remains in a shockable rhythm, the second and subsequent shocks should be at 4 J/kg. Amiodarone should be considered after the second unsuccessful shock. Transport as soon as possible.

Pulseless Electrical Activity. The patient with PEA is pulseless and apneic. Resuscitation should be directed toward correcting the underlying cause. Otherwise, treatment is the same as for asystole.

Neurologic Emergencies
pp. 116–117

Seizures. When confronted with a seizing child, determine whether there is a history of seizures or seizures with fever. Also, determine how many seizures occurred during the incident. If the child is not seizing upon your arrival, elicit a description of the seizure activity. Note the condition and position of the child when found. Question parents, caregivers, or bystanders about the possibility of head injury. A history of irritability or lethargy prior to the seizure may indicate CNS infection. If possible, find out whether the child suffers from diabetes or has recently complained of a headache or a stiff neck. Note any current medications, as well as possible ingestions. The physical examination should be systematic. Pay particular attention to the adequacy of respirations, the level of consciousness, neurologic evaluation, and signs of injury. Also inspect the child for signs of dehydration. Dehydration may be evidenced by the absence of tears or, in an infant, by the presence of a sunken fontanelle.

Management of pediatric seizures is essentially the same as for seizing adults. Place patients on the floor or on the bed. Be sure to lay them on their side, away from the furniture. Do not restrain patients, but take steps to protect them from injury. Maintain the airway, but do not force anything, such as a bite stick, between the teeth. Administer supplemental oxygen if the patient is hypoxic. Then take and record all vital signs. If the patient is febrile, remove excess layers of clothing, while avoiding extreme cooling. If status epilepticus is present, institute the following steps: start an IV of normal saline or lactated Ringer's and perform a glucometer evaluation; administer diazepam or lorazepam as directed; contact medical direction for additional dosing. If the seizure appears to be caused by fever and a long transport time is anticipated, medical direction may request the administration of acetaminophen to lower the fever. Acetaminophen is supplied as an elixir or as suppositories. The dose should be 15 mg/kg body weight. Transport. Reassure and support the parents or caregivers, as this is a very stressful and frightening situation for them.

Meningitis. Meningitis is more common in children than in adults. Findings in the history that may suggest meningitis include a child who has been ill for one day to several days, a recent ear or respiratory tract infection, high fever, lethargy or irritability, a severe headache, or a stiff neck. Infants generally do not develop a stiff neck. They will generally become lethargic and will not feed well. Some babies may simply develop a fever. On physical examination, the child with meningitis will appear very ill. With an infant, the fontanelle may be bulging or full unless accompanied by dehydration. Extreme discomfort with movement, owing to irritation of the meninges, may be present.

Prehospital care of the pediatric patient with meningitis is supportive. Complete the primary assessment rapidly and transport the child to the emergency department. If shock is present, treat the child with intravenous fluids (20 mL/kg) and oxygen.

Nausea and Vomiting. Treatment of pediatric nausea and vomiting is primarily supportive. If the child is dehydrated and unable to keep oral fluids down, intravenous fluid therapy may be indicated. Severe dehydration, as evidenced by prolonged capillary refill time, should be treated with 20-mL/kg fluid boluses of lactated Ringer's solution or 0.9 percent sodium chloride solution (normal saline).

Diarrhea. Treatment of the child suffering from diarrhea is primarily supportive. If dehydration is evident, administer fluids. Oral hydration works quite well. Severe dehydration should be treated with 20-mL/kg boluses of intravenous fluids (lactated Ringer's or normal saline).

Diabetic Emergencies pp. 118–119

Hypoglycemia. Measure blood glucose with a glucometer and elicit a history of conditions known to cause hypoglycemia in infants and children. Treatment should be initiated whenever you have a high index of suspicion and/or blood sugar drops below 70 mg/dL (≤ 3.9 mmol/L). Signs and symptoms of moderate hypoglycemia include sweating, tremors, irritability, vomiting, mood swings, blurred vision, stomachache, headache, dizziness, and slurred speech. Signs and symptoms of severe hypoglycemia include decreased level of consciousness, seizures, tachycardia, and hypoperfusion.

In the conscious, alert patient, administer oral fluids with sugar or oral glucose per medical direction. If there is no response, or if the patient exhibits an altered mental status, transport immediately. Consult your medical direction physician on orders for the administration of dextrose or intramuscular (IM) glucagon. Twenty-five percent dextrose solution ($D_{25}W$) can be prepared by diluting 50 percent dextrose solution 1:1 with sterile water or saline. A 10 percent dextrose solution ($D_{10}W$) will also work. It is easier to dose children with this concentration, and it does not cause as much discomfort as with intravenous administration. Repeat blood glucose tests within 10 to 15 minutes of infusion or the administration of glucose. In treating diabetic pediatric patients, remember that most children have been taught about their condition and can participate, in varying degrees, in their care.

Hyperglycemia. In cases of hyperglycemia, glucose is spilled into the urine, taking water with it through osmotic diuresis. This can result in a significant fluid loss with resultant dehydration. Keep in mind that acidosis results from the accumulation of ketones, a by-product of fat metabolism. A continual increase in the ketones eventually leads to metabolic acidosis, which produces the fruity breath odor commonly associated with hyperglycemia. Signs and symptoms of late hyperglycemia include weakness, abdominal pain, generalized aches, loss of appetite, nausea and vomiting, signs of dehydration (except increased urine output), fruity breath odor, tachypnea, hyperventilation, and tachycardia. Signs and symptoms of ketoacidosis include continued decreased level of consciousness progressing to coma, Kussmaul's respirations, and signs of dehydration. A blood sugar reading of greater than 200 mg/dL typically indicates hyperglycemia.

Carefully monitor the ABCs and vital signs. If you cannot confirm the presence of hyperglycemia with a blood glucose test, consider administering oral fluids with sugar or oral glucose in case the patient is hypoglycemic. If intravenous access is possible, consider initiating an IV of either normal saline or lactated Ringer's. Administer an IV bolus of 20 mL/kg, and repeat the bolus if the patient's vital signs do not change. Monitor the patient's mental status and be prepared to intubate if the respirations continue to decrease. Remember, this is a potentially life-threatening situation. Consult with medical direction on all actions taken and transport immediately.

Poisoning and Toxicologic Emergencies pp. 119–121

Poisoning can cause many different signs and symptoms, depending on the poison ingested, the route of exposure, and the time since exposure. Narcotics and some of the hydrocarbons can cause respiratory system depression. Digitalis, beta-blockers, calcium-channel blockers, and many of the antihypertensive agents can cause circulatory depression or collapse. A great many agents can impair the central nervous system. These include alcohol, barbiturates, narcotics, and cocaine. Virtually any substance can affect thought and behavior. Common agents are the anticholinergics, alcohol, narcotics, hydrocarbons, and many others. Aspirin, corrosives, and hydrocarbons can irritate or destroy the gastrointestinal system. Acetaminophen can cause liver necrosis and, eventually, liver failure.

General steps in managing a responsive pediatric poisoning patient include the following: administer oxygen (if the patient is hypoxic), contact medical direction and/or the poison control center, consider the need for activated charcoal, transport (be sure to take any pills, substances, and containers to the hospital), and monitor the patient continuously in case the child suddenly becomes unresponsive.

General steps in managing an unresponsive pediatric poisoning patient include the following: ensure a patent airway, suction if necessary, administer oxygen (if the patient is hypoxic), be prepared to provide artificial ventilations if respiratory failure or cardiac arrest is present, contact medical direction and/or the poison control center, transport (be sure to take any pills, substances, and containers to the hospital), monitor the patient continuously, and rule out trauma as a cause of altered mental status.

Trauma
pp. 121–126

Traumatic Brain Injury. Traumatic head injuries can cause intracranial bleeding or swelling. This ultimately results in an increase in intracranial pressure. The signs of increased intracranial pressure can be subtle and include elevated blood pressure; bradycardia; rapid, deep respirations progressing to slow, deep respirations; and bulging fontanelle in infants. Increased intracranial pressure will eventually lead to herniation of a portion of the brain through the foramen magnum. This is an ominous development that is often associated with irreversible injury. Signs and symptoms of herniation include asymmetrical pupils, decorticate posturing and decerebrate posturing.

Specific management of traumatic head injuries in children is similar to that for adults. As a rule, follow these steps: administer supplemental oxygen (if the patient is hypoxic); provide ventilation, consider intubation in children with a Glasgow coma score of less than or equal to 8 (severe head injury) and ventilate at a normal rate; and consider rapid sequence intubation (RSI) for children with a Glasgow coma score of less than or equal to 8 who have too much muscle tone to allow endotracheal intubation.

Consider hyperventilation only if there is a deterioration in the child's condition as evidenced by asymmetric pupils, active seizures, or neurologic posturing (indicating herniation). Children with traumatic head injuries do best at facilities that treat a great number of children and who have pediatric neurosurgeons on staff. Consider diverting to a pediatric trauma facility if a moderate or severe traumatic head injury is present.

Head, Face, and Neck. In treating head injuries, remember that diffuse injuries are common in children, whereas focal injuries are rare. Because the skull is softer and more compliant in children than in adults, brain injuries occur more readily in infants and young children. Because of open fontanelles and sutures, infants up to an average age of 16 months may be more tolerant to an increase in intracranial pressure and can have delayed signs. (Keep this fact in mind when taking the history of children in the 1-month-to-2-years age range.)

Injuries to the Chest. Because of the compliance of the chest wall, severe intrathoracic injury can be present without signs of external injury. Tension pneumothorax presents with the following signs and symptoms: diminished breath sounds over the affected lung, shift of the trachea to the opposite side, and progressive decrease in ventilatory compliance. Keep in mind that children with cardiac tamponade may have no physical signs of tamponade other than hypotension. Also remember that flail chest is an uncommon injury in children. When chest injury is noted without a significant mechanism of injury, suspect child abuse.

Injuries to the Abdomen. Signs and symptoms of a splenic injury include tenderness in the left upper quadrant of the abdomen, abrasions on the abdomen, and hematoma of the abdominal wall. Symptoms of liver injury include right upper quadrant abdominal pain and/or right lower chest pain. In treating blunt abdominal trauma, keep in mind the small size of the pediatric abdomen. Be certain to palpate only one quadrant at a time. In cases of both chest and abdominal trauma, treat for shock with positioning, fluids, and maintenance of body temperature.

Extremities. Whenever indicated, perform splinting in order to decrease pain and prevent further injury and/or blood loss.

Drowning
pp. 122–123

As with the other injury processes, the best treatment is prevention. EMS personnel, in conjunction with local building inspectors, can inspect pools for safety. A pool should be fenced off with a gate that closes automatically. Essential rescue equipment (pole, life preserver) should be immediately available and the local emergency number posted. The best time for drowning prevention programs is late spring and early summer. Encourage parents to enroll their children in water safety classes as early as possible.

Burns

pp. 123; 126–127

Estimation of the burn surface area is slightly different for children than for adults. In a child, the head accounts for a larger percentage of body surface area (BSA), whereas the legs make up a smaller percentage. Thus, for children the rule of nines is modified to take away 8 percent from the lower extremities (2 percent from the front and 2 percent from the back of each leg) plus the 1 percent assigned to the adult genitalia. This 9 percent that is taken from the lower part of the body is reassigned to the head. Therefore, whereas the adult's entire head and neck are counted as 9 percent, in the child the anterior head and neck count as 9 percent and the posterior head and neck count as another 9 percent. You can also use the child's palm as a guide (the "rule of palm"). The palm equals about 1 percent of the body surface area. You can calculate a burn area by estimating how many palm areas it equals. Usually, the rule of nines works best for more extensive burns and the rule of palm for less extensive ones.

Management considerations for pediatric burn patients include the following: provide prompt management of the airway, because swelling can develop rapidly; if intubation is required, you may need to use an endotracheal tube up to two sizes smaller than normal because of the swelling; thermally burned children are very susceptible to hypothermia, so be sure to maintain body heat; and when treating serious electrical burn patients, suspect musculoskeletal injuries and perform spinal immobilization.

10. **Adapt equipment and techniques of management to meet the needs of pediatric patients in positioning and immobilization, airway management, ventilation, oxygenation, vascular access, fluid and medication administration, and cardiac arrest management.** pp. 89–105

Manual Positioning. Allow the pediatric patient to assume a position of comfort, if possible. When placing the patient in a supine position, avoid hyperextension of the neck. For trauma patients less than 3 years old, place support under the torso. For supine medical patients 3 years old and older, provide occipital elevation.

Foreign Body Airway Obstruction. Avoid any maneuvers that will turn a mild obstruction into a severe obstruction. Instead, place the patient in a position of comfort and transport immediately. For children older than 1 year of age, perform a series of abdominal thrusts until the item is expelled or the victim becomes unresponsive. If the victim becomes unresponsive, start CPR. For an infant, deliver a series of five back blows followed by five chest thrusts (abdominal thrusts are not recommended for infants). Inspect the infant's mouth on completion of each series. If the infant becomes unresponsive, begin CPR.

If a child's airway cannot be cleared by basic airway procedures, visualize the airway with the laryngoscope. Often, the obstructing foreign body can be seen. Once it is visualized, grasp the foreign body with Magill forceps and remove it. If you cannot remove the foreign body with Magill forceps, try to intubate around the obstruction. This often requires using an endotracheal tube smaller than you would normally choose. However, this will provide an adequate airway until the foreign body can be removed at the hospital. Finally, if the foreign body cannot be removed with Magill forceps and it is impossible to intubate around it, then you should consider placing a cricothyrotomy needle. This should only be done as a last resort. Be sure to follow local protocols regarding needle cricothyrotomy.

Suctioning. Apply suctioning whenever you detect heavy secretions in the nose or mouth of a pediatric patient, especially if the patient has a diminished level of consciousness. You can use a bulb syringe, flexible suction catheter, or rigid-tip suction catheter, depending on the patient's age or size. Make sure that flexible catheters are correctly sized. Although pediatric suctioning techniques vary very little from adult suctioning techniques, keep the following modifications in mind: decrease suction pressure to less than 100 mmHg in infants; avoid excessive suctioning time (suction less than 10 seconds) in order to decrease the possibility of hypoxia; and avoid stimulation of the vagus nerve, which may produce bradycardia. Frequently check the patient's pulse; if bradycardia occurs, stop suctioning immediately and oxygenate.

Oxygenation. When possible, use pulse oximetry to guide supplemental oxygen administration. The goal is to provide just enough oxygen to maintain a SpO_2 of 94 percent or greater. For resuscitation, use 100 percent oxygen when possible (except in newborns). Methods of oxygen delivery include "blow-by" techniques (especially for neonates) and pediatric-sized nonrebreather masks. If the child refuses to accept the nonrebreather mask, resort to high-concentration blow-by oxygen.

Oropharyngeal Airways. Oropharyngeal airways should be used only in pediatric patients who lack a gag reflex. Size the airway by measuring from the corner of the mouth to the front of the earlobe. In placing an oropharyngeal airway, use a tongue blade to depress the tongue and jaw. If you detect a gag reflex, continue to maintain an open airway with a manual (head-tilt/chin-lift) maneuver and consider the use of a nasal airway. Remember that with a pediatric patient, the oral airway is inserted with the tip pointing toward the tongue and pharynx.

Nasopharyngeal Airways. Use nasopharyngeal airways for those children who possess a gag reflex and who require prolonged artificial ventilations. Do not use them on any child with midface or head trauma. Size a nasal airway by using the outside diameter of the patient's little finger as a measure. Although nasopharyngeal airways come in a variety of sizes, they are not readily available for infants less than 1 year old. When inserting the nasal airway, follow the same basic method as you would in an adult patient. It is important to remember that younger children often have enlarged adenoids (lymphatic tissues in the nasopharynx), which can be easily lacerated when inserting a nasopharyngeal airway. Because of this, always use care when inserting a nasopharyngeal airway in a younger child. If resistance is met, do not force the airway because significant bleeding can result.

Ventilation. Ventilation is a two-way physiologic street: Maintenance of appropriate oxygen levels results in appropriate carbon dioxide levels as well. However, you will achieve neither of these clinically important events without tailoring the ventilatory device and technique to your pediatric patient. Important points to remember include the following: avoid excessive bag pressure and volume (hyperventilation); ventilate at an age-appropriate rate, using only enough ventilation to make the chest rise; use continuous waveform capnography to monitor and guide ventilation; use a properly sized mask to ensure a good fit; flow-restricted, oxygen-powered ventilation devices are contraindicated in pediatric resuscitation; do not use BVMs with pop-off valves unless they can be readily occluded, if necessary; apply cricoid pressure to minimize gastric inflation and passive regurgitation in unresponsive children; avoid excessive cricoid pressure so as not to obstruct the trachea; and ensure correct positioning to avoid hyperextension of the neck.

Needle Cricothyrotomy. Needle cricothyrotomy in children is the same as in adult patients. It is important to remember that the anatomic landmarks are smaller and more difficult to identify. Remember, the only indication for cricothyrotomy is failure to obtain an airway by any other method.

Endotracheal Intubation. Pediatric endotracheal intubation has come under increasing scrutiny in EMS. Several studies have questioned the effectiveness of prehospital pediatric endotracheal intubation. Bag-mask ventilation can be as effective, and may be safer, than endotracheal tube ventilation for short periods during prehospital resuscitation. Although endotracheal intubation of a child and an adult follow the same basic procedures, the special features of the pediatric airway complicate placement of any orotracheal tube. In fact, variations in the airway size of children preclude the use of certain airways, including esophageal obturator airways (EOAs), pharyngeotracheal lumen airways (PtLs), and esophageal tracheal Combitubes (ETCs). Properly sized laryngeal mask airways (LMAs) may be used in children but do not protect the airway from aspiration.

In infants and small children, it is often more difficult to create a single clear visual plane from the mouth, through the pharynx, and into the glottis. A straight-blade laryngoscope is preferred, as it provides greater displacement of the tongue and better visualization of the relatively cephalad and anterior glottis. For larger children, a curved blade may sometimes be used. Variations in the sizes of pediatric airways, coupled with the fact that the narrowest portion of the airway is at the level of the cricoid ring, make proper sizing of the endotracheal tube crucial. To determine correct size, apply any of the following methods: use a resuscitation tape, such as the Broselow™ tape, to estimate tube size based on height; estimate the correct tube size by using the diameter of the patient's little finger or the diameter of the nasal opening; or calculate the correct tube size by using this simple numerical formula: (Patient's age in years + 16) ÷ 4 = Tube size. The best method of determining depth is direct visualization. Because of the distance between the mouth and the trachea, a stylet is rarely needed to position the tube properly. When a stylet is used, select a malleable yet rigid style. Either cuffed or uncuffed endotracheal tubes can be used in children (but not in neonates). In certain conditions, a cuffed tube may be superior, but cuff pressure should be limited to 20 cm H_2O. Infants and small children may have greater vagal response than adults. Therefore, laryngoscopy and passage of an endotracheal tube are likely to cause a vagal response, dramatically slowing the child's heart rate and decreasing the cardiac output and blood pressure. As a result, pediatric intubations must be carried out swiftly, accurately, and with continuous monitoring. As with adults, allow no more than 30 seconds to pass without ventilating your patient.

You must always verify and document proper endotracheal tube placement and ensure that the tube remains properly situated in the trachea throughout care. Proper endotracheal tube placement can be determined by several methods. First, the paramedic performing the intubation should see the tube pass between the cords. Second, bilateral chest rise should be observed with mechanical ventilation and breath sounds over the epigastrium should be absent. The presence of condensation on the inside of the endotracheal tube also suggests proper tube placement. Additionally, the lack of phonation (vocal sounds) indicates that the tube is properly placed into the trachea. Esophageal detector devices are sometimes used in prehospital care to confirm proper tube placement. However, it is important to use these devices with caution in pediatric patients because you might get a false-positive finding even if the tube is improperly placed. This is particularly true when uncuffed endotracheal tubes have been used. The preferred method of endotracheal tube verification is through the use of capnography with either a colorimetric detector or waveform capnography.

It is not uncommon for an endotracheal tube to become displaced during patient care, movement, or transport. Because of this, paramedics must be extremely vigilant about repeatedly or continuously monitoring proper endotracheal tube placement. Monitoring can be accomplished through repeated assessments or through the use of continuous waveform capnography. Continuous waveform capnography provides breath-to-breath verification of proper tube placement and will rapidly alert providers of a problem with ventilation or with endotracheal tube placement.

Extraglottic Airways. The laryngeal mask airway (LMA) is now routinely used in several EMS systems for prehospital airway management. The LMA is easy to insert and requires less education and practice than endotracheal intubation.

Nasogastric Intubation. If gastric distention is present in a pediatric patient, you may consider placing a nasogastric (NG) tube. An NG tube can also be used to empty the stomach of blood or other substances. In sizing the NG tube, keep in mind the following recommended guidelines: newborn/infant (8.0 french), toddler/preschooler (10 french), school-age children (12 french), and adolescents (14–16 french). In determining the correct length, measure the tube from the tip of the nose, over the ear, to the tip of the xiphoid process.

Vascular Access. Intravenous techniques for children are basically the same as for adults. However, additional veins may be accessed in the infant. These include veins of the neck and scalp as well as those of the arms, hands, and feet. The external jugular vein, however, should be used only for life-threatening situations.

Intraosseous Infusion. The use of intraosseous (IO) infusion has become popular in treating pediatric patients. Certain medications can be administered intraosseously, including epinephrine, atropine, dopamine, lidocaine, sodium bicarbonate, and dobutamine. Several of the intraosseous devices, such as the EZ-IO® and the Bone Injection Gun (B.I.G.), are approved for usage in children.

Fluid Therapy. The primary dosage of fluid in hypovolemic shock should be 20 mL/kg of an isotonic solution such as lactated Ringer's or normal saline as soon as IV access is obtained. After the infusion, the child should be reassessed. If perfusion is still diminished, then a second bolus of 20 mL/kg should be administered. A child with hypovolemic shock may require 40 to 60 mL/kg, whereas a child with septic shock may require at least 60 to 80 mL/kg. Fluid therapy should be guided by the child's clinical response.

Medications. Cardiopulmonary arrest in infants and children is almost always the result of a primary respiratory problem, such as drowning, choking, or smoke inhalation. The major aim in pediatric resuscitation is airway management and ventilation, as well as replacement of intravascular volume, if

©2013 Pearson Education, Inc.
Paramedic Care: Principles & Practice, Vol. 6, 4th Ed.

indicated. In certain cases, medications may be required. The dosages of medications must be modified for the pediatric patient. Use a resuscitation tape, such as the Broselow™ tape, to show recommended pediatric drug dosages.

Electrical Therapy. You are less likely to use electrical therapy on pediatric patients than on adult patients, because ventricular fibrillation is much less common in children than adults. However, you should review and keep the following principles in mind for times when these emergencies arise:

- Administer an initial dosage of 2 to 4 joules per kilogram of body weight. (Keep in mind the estimated body weights in Table 4–5.)
- If this is unsuccessful, focus your attention on correcting hypoxia and acidosis.
- Transport to a pediatric critical care unit, if possible.

C-Spine Immobilization. Spinal injuries in children are not as common as in adults. However, because of a child's disproportionately larger and heavier head, the cervical spine (C-spine) is vulnerable to injury. Always make sure that you use the appropriate-sized pediatric immobilization equipment. These supplies may include rigid cervical collars, towel or blanket rolls, foam head blocks, commercial pediatric immobilization devices, vest-type or short wooden backboards, and long boards with the appropriate padding. For pediatric patients found in car seats, you can also use the seat for immobilization. The Kendrick extrication device (KED) can be quickly modified to immobilize a pediatric patient.

11. Recognize indications of abuse or neglect of a pediatric patient.   pp. 128–129

Child abuse can take several forms, including psychological abuse, physical abuse, sexual abuse, and physical or emotional neglect. Abused children suffer every imaginable kind of mistreatment. They are battered with fists, belts, broom handles, hairbrushes, baseball bats, electric cords, and any other objects that can be used as weapons. They are locked in closets, denied food, or deprived of access to a toilet. They are intentionally burned or scalded with anything from hot water to cigarette butts to open flames. They are severely shaken, thrown into cribs, pushed down stairs, or shoved into walls. Some are shot, stabbed, or suffocated. Sexual abuse ranges from adults exposing themselves to children to overt sexual acts to sexual torture.

Signs of abuse or neglect can be startling. As a guide, the following findings should trigger a high index of suspicion: any obvious or suspected fractures in a child under 2 years of age; multiple injuries in various stages of healing, especially burns and bruises; more injuries than usually seen in children of the same age or size; injuries scattered on many areas of the body; bruises or burns in patterns that suggest intentional infliction; increased intracranial pressure in an infant; suspected intra-abdominal trauma in a young child; and any injury that does not fit with the description of the cause given.

Information in the medical history may also raise the index of suspicion. Examples include a history that does not match the nature or severity of the injury; vague parental accounts or accounts that change during the interview; accusations that the child injured himself intentionally; delay in seeking help; child dressed inappropriately for the situation; and revealing comments by bystanders, especially siblings.

Suspect child neglect if you spot any of the following conditions: extreme malnutrition, multiple insect bites, long-standing skin infections, extreme lack of cleanliness, verbal or social skills far below those you would expect for a child of similar age and background, or lack of appropriate medical care.

12. Describe special considerations in management and documentation of situations involving SIDS, ALTE, abuse, and neglect.   pp. 127–129

Sudden infant death syndrome (SIDS) is defined as the sudden death of an infant during the first year of life from an illness of unknown etiology. The immediate needs of the family with a SIDS baby are many. Unless the infant is obviously dead, undertake active and aggressive care of the infant to assure the family that everything possible is being done. A first responder or other personnel should be assigned to assist the parents and to explain the procedures. At all points, use the baby's name. After arrival at the hospital, direct management at the parents or caregivers, as nothing can be done for the child. Allow the family to see the dead child. Expect a normal grief reaction. Initially, there may be shock, disbelief, and denial. Other times, the parents or caregivers may express anger, rage, hostility, blame, or guilt. Often, there is a feeling of inadequacy as well as helplessness, confusion, and fear. The grief process is likely to last for years. SIDS has major long-term effects on family relations. It may also affect you, the on-scene paramedic. If so, do not be reluctant to seek counseling.

The term *apparent life-threatening event* (ALTE) is defined as a sudden event, often characterized by apnea or other abrupt changes in the child's behavior. These episodes may necessitate stimulation or resuscitation to arouse the child and reinitiate regular breathing. ALTE was once referred to as "near near-miss SIDS." From an EMS standpoint, the care provided should be based upon your assessment and immediate life threats.

A tragic truth is that some people cause physical and psychological harm to children, either through intentional abuse or through intentional or unintentional neglect. The person who abuses or neglects a child can come from any geographic, religious, ethnic, racial, occupational, educational, or socioeconomic background. Despite their diversity, people who abuse children tend to share certain traits: a parent or adult who seems capable of abuse, especially one who exhibits evasive or hostile behavior; a child in one of the high-risk categories; or the presence of a crisis, particularly financial stress, marital or relationship stress, or physical illness in a parent or child.

In cases of child abuse or neglect, the goals of management include appropriate treatment of injuries, protection of the child from further abuse, and notification of proper authorities. You should obtain as much information as possible, in a nonjudgmental manner. Document all findings or statements in the patient report. Do not "cross-examine" the parents. Try to be supportive toward the parents, especially if it helps you to transport the child to the hospital. Remember: Never leave transport to the alleged abuser. Upon arrival at the emergency department, report your suspicions to the appropriate personnel. Complete the patient report and all available documentation at this time, as delay may inhibit accurate recall of data. Child abuse and neglect are particularly stressful aspects of emergency medical services. You must recognize and deal with your feelings, perhaps by seeking counseling.

13. Work with caregivers to troubleshoot home care equipment for special needs pediatric patients and intervene as needed.   pp. 129–132

Devices you might commonly find in the home include tracheostomy tubes, apnea monitors, home artificial ventilators, central intravenous lines, gastric feeding tubes, gastrostomy tubes, and shunts. In treating children with special needs, remember that the parents and caregivers are often very knowledgeable about their children and the devices that sustain their lives. Listen to them.

A tracheostomy tube may be used as a temporary or a permanent device. Although various types of tubes are used, you might encounter some common complications, including obstruction, site bleeding, air leakage, dislodged tube, or infection. Care steps involve maintaining an open airway, suctioning the tube, allowing the patient to remain in a position of comfort, administering oxygen in cases of respiratory distress, assisting ventilations in cases of respiratory failure/arrest, and transporting the patient to the hospital.

Apnea monitors are used to alert parents or caregivers to the cessation of breathing in an infant, especially a premature infant. If the device does not detect a breath within a specific time frame or if the infant's heart rate is too slow or too fast, an alarm will sound. When an apnea monitor is placed in a home, the parents are typically instructed on what to do if the alarm sounds (stimulate the child, provide artificial respirations, and so on). If these fail, EMS may be summoned. Also, nervous parents who have just brought a baby home on an apnea monitor may panic the first couple of times the alarm sounds and call 911. Be patient and kind while instructing them on what to do when the alarm sounds.

Various configurations exist for home ventilators. Demand ventilators sense the rate and quality of a patient's respiration as well as several other parameters, including pulse oximetry. They typically respond to preset limits. Other devices provide a constant positive end-expiratory pressure (PEEP) and a set oxygen concentration for the patient. Two complications commonly result in EMS calls: a device's mechanical failure and shortages of energy during an electrical failure. Care steps involve maintaining an open airway, administering artificial ventilations via an appropriately sized BVM with oxygen, and transporting the patient to a hospital until the home ventilator is working.

Children who require long-term IV therapy will often have central lines placed into the superior vena cava near the heart. If IV therapy is only necessary for several weeks, percutaneous intravenous catheter (PIC) lines may be placed in the arm and threaded into the superior vena cava. Central IV lines are commonly used to administer intravenous nutrition, antibiotics, or chemotherapy for cancer. Possible complications for central IV lines include cracked line, infection, loss of patency, hemorrhage, and air embolism. Care steps involve control of any bleeding through direct pressure. If a large amount of air is in the line, try to withdraw it with a syringe. If this fails, clamp the line and transport. In cases of a

©2013 Pearson Education, Inc.
Paramedic Care: Principles & Practice, Vol. 6, 4th Ed.

cracked line, place a clamp between the crack and the patient. If the patient exhibits an altered mental status following the cracked line, position the child on the left side with head down. Transport the child to the hospital as quickly as possible.

Children who are not capable of swallowing or eating receive nutrition through either a gastric feeding tube (placed through the abdominal wall into the stomach) or a gastrostomy tube (placed through the nostrils into the stomach). These special devices are commonly used in disorders of the digestive system or in situations in which the developmental ability of the patient hinders feeding. Possible emergency complications include bleeding at the site, dislodged tube, and respiratory distress. Care steps involve supporting the ABCs, including possible suctioning and administration of supplemental oxygen. Patients should be transported to a definitive care facility, either in a sitting position or lying on the right side with the head elevated. The goal is to reduce the risk of aspiration, a serious condition.

A shunt is a surgical connection that runs from the brain to the abdomen. It removes excess cerebrospinal fluid from the brain through drainage. Cases of shunt failure present as altered mental status. The patient may exhibit drowsiness, respiratory distress, or the classic signs of pupil dysfunction or posturing. Care steps involve maintenance of an open airway, administration of ventilations as needed, and immediate transport.

14. Apply the JumpSTART triage method to multiple-casualty incidents involving children. pp. 132–133

The JumpSTART Pediatric MCI Triage Tool is an objective tool developed specifically for the triage of children in the multicasualty/disaster setting. The steps of the JumpSTART system are:

1. **Identify and direct all ambulatory patients to designated minor (GREEN) area for secondary triage and treatment.** Begin assessment of nonambulatory patients as you come to them. Because children less than 1 year of age cannot walk, they should be carried to the minor (GREEN) area by other ambulatory victims and must be the first assessed by medical personnel in that area.
2. **Assess breathing.** If the child is breathing spontaneously, go on to the next step (assessing respiratory rate). If the child is apneic or with very irregular breathing, open the airway using standard positioning techniques. If positioning results in resumption of spontaneous respirations, tag the patient immediate (RED) and move on. If the child is not breathing after airway opening, check for peripheral pulse. If no pulse, tag the patient deceased/nonsalvageable (BLACK) and move on. If there is a peripheral pulse, give 5 mouth-to-barrier ventilations. If apnea persists, tag the patient deceased/nonsalvageable (BLACK) and move on. If breathing resumes after the "jumpstart" (ventilation attempt), tag the patient immediate (RED) and move on.
3. **Assess respiratory rate.** If the child's respiratory rate is 15 to 45 per minute, proceed to the next step (assess perfusion). If respiratory rate is < 15 or > 45 per minute or irregular, tag patient as immediate (RED) and move on.
4. **Assess perfusion.** If a peripheral pulse is palpable, proceed to the next step (assess mental status). If no peripheral pulse is present (in the least injured limb), tag the patient immediate (RED) and move on.
5. **Assess mental status.** Use the AVPU scale to assess mental status. If the patient is alert, responsive to verbal stimuli, or appropriately responsive to pain, tag as delayed (YELLOW) and move on. If the patient is inappropriately responsive to pain or is unresponsive, tag as immediate (RED) and move on.

Unless clearly suffering from injuries incompatible with life, victims tagged in the dead/nonsalvageable (BLACK) category should be reassessed once critical interventions have been completed for immediate (RED) and delayed (YELLOW) patients. Care should be taken to preserve the dignity of the dead, at the same time being careful to not disturb any forensic evidence present.

15. Communicate relevant patient information orally and in writing when transferring care of the pediatric patient to hospital personnel. pp. 72–133

During your classroom, clinical, and field training, you will interact and communicate with real and simulated patients, family members, bystanders, other responders, and hospital personnel. Pediatric emergencies can be stressful for both you and the adults responsible for the child's well-being. In addition to the information presented in this chapter, you will use the information from Volume 1, Chapter 9: EMS System Communications; Volume 1, Chapter 10: Documentation; and Volume 3, Chapter 3:

Therapeutic Communications to effectively communicate and document assessment findings, patient management, and patient response to care. Continue to refine these skills once your training ends and you begin your career as a paramedic.

Case Study Review

Reread the case study on page 71 in Paramedic Care: Special Patients; *then, read the following discussion.*

This case study examines the treatment of a severely dehydrated pediatric patient—a common condition encountered on calls involving infants and young children.

This case involves an infant who has been unable to hold down any food for three days. In just a short time, she has developed signs and symptoms that point to possible shock, which the paramedics immediately notice. Their initial assessment starts as soon they observe the quality of the baby's skin (pale, cool, clammy) and the noticeably sunken anterior fontanelle. As the paramedics take vital signs and assess the level of consciousness, they note that the baby cries but does not produce tears. After taking appropriate Standard Precautions, they wisely check the infant's diaper to see if it is dry or wet. (If it had been wet, they would have checked the quality of the urine. Dehydrated patients, when they do urinate, have very dark yellow urine because it is a concentrated solute with less solvent [water] than usual.) The dry diaper and the mother's comment confirms a suspicion of dehydration, giving the crew enough information to develop a treatment plan.

The paramedics take this patient very seriously and begin transport before starting fluid therapy. En route to the hospital, they start an IV, which is not always an easy task in a patient this small. They probably keep in mind the use of an intraosseous needle in case an IV cannot be placed. For a patient this dehydrated, it would not be surprising that she might have needed a second bolus of 20 mL/kg of the normal saline. Of course, as is always the case, a parent should be nearby to assist in comforting the patient.

During your paramedic career, you can expect to take part in a call similar to this one. Dehydration in infants and small children is a common condition, and you should be prepared to respond, assess, and manage the patient accordingly. Remember that dehydration is one of the causes of hypoperfusion (shock) in pediatric patients.

Content Self-Evaluation

MULTIPLE CHOICE

_____ 1. The leading cause of death in pediatric patients in the United States is
    A. AIDS.
    B. asthma.
    C. trauma.
    D. neglect.
    E. cardiac arrest.

_____ 2. Factors that account for high rates of pediatric injury include all of the following, EXCEPT
    A. weather.
    B. geography.
    C. dangers in the home.
    D. decreased requirements for seat belt usage.
    E. motor vehicle accidents.

_____ 3. The federally funded program aimed at improving the health of pediatric patients who suffer from life-threatening illnesses and injuries is called
    A. EMSC.
    B. PEPP.
    C. PALS.
    D. APLS.
    E. TRIPP.

©2013 Pearson Education, Inc.
Paramedic Care: Principles & Practice, Vol. 6, 4th Ed.

_____ **4.** Treatment of a pediatric patient begins with
 A. obtaining vital signs.
 B. placement of an ET tube.
 C. administration of oxygen.
 D. focused head-to-toe exam.
 E. communications and psychological support.

_____ **5.** The most common response of children to illness or injury is
 A. denial.   D. indifference.
 B. fear.   E. grief.
 C. excitement.

_____ **6.** While caring for the pediatric patient, whenever possible, the paramedic should
 A. avoid discussing painful procedures.
 B. administer high-concentration oxygen.
 C. allow a parent or caregiver to stay with the child.
 D. use correct medical and anatomical terms.
 E. stand in an authoritative posture.

_____ **7.** The term *neonate* describes a baby who is
 A. newly born.   D. 1 to 5 months in age.
 B. 10 days or less in age.   E. 6 months or more in age.
 C. up to 1 month in age.

_____ **8.** The age group for which foreign body airway obstruction (FBAO) first becomes a concern is
 A. infants, ages 1–5 months.   D. preschoolers.
 B. infants, ages 6–12 months. E. school-age children.
 C. toddlers.

_____ **9.** An infant's airway differs from that of an adult in all of the following ways, EXCEPT that it
 A. is narrower at all levels.
 B. has a softer and more flexible trachea.
 C. is less likely to be blocked by secretions.
 D. has a greater likelihood of soft tissue injury.
 E. is more prone to obstruction by the tongue.

_____ **10.** Unlike an adult, the trachea of a child can collapse if the neck and head are hyperextended because
 A. the trachea is softer and more flexible.
 B. a child's tongue takes up more space proportionately.
 C. the cricoid rings are firmer.
 D. a child's larynx is higher.
 E. the airway is wider at all levels.

_____ **11.** The two abdominal organs that are most likely to suffer traumatic injury in a pediatric patient are the
 A. kidney and gallbladder.   D. colon and appendix.
 B. liver and spleen.   E. bladder and pancreas.
 C. stomach and small intestine.

_____ **12.** A child's larger BSA-to-weight ratio causes a pediatric patient to be
 A. resilient to temperature changes.
 B. prone to hypothermia.
 C. difficult to assess.
 D. prone to excess subcutaneous fat.
 E. less likely to lose fluids quickly.

13. Although infants and children have a circulating blood volume proportionately larger than that of adults, their absolute blood volume is
    A. about the same.
    B. smaller.
    C. even larger.
    D. rate dependent.
    E. variable.

14. The pediatric assessment triangle focuses on airway, breathing, and circulation.
    A. True
    B. False

15. In an infant or small child, tachypnea, an abnormally rapid rate of breathing, may indicate
    A. fear.
    B. pain.
    C. inadequate oxygenation.
    D. exposure to cold.
    E. all of the above.

16. In comparing pediatric heart and respiratory rates with those of an adult, infants and young children have
    A. about the same heart and respiratory rates as an adult.
    B. slower heart rates and slower respiratory rates than an adult.
    C. slower heart rates and faster respiratory rates than an adult.
    D. faster heart rates and slower respiratory rates than an adult.
    E. faster heart rates and faster respiratory rates than an adult.

17. A respiratory rate of 18 to 30 breaths per minute would be considered normal for a
    A. newborn.
    B. 6-month-old infant.
    C. toddler.
    D. preschooler.
    E. school-age child.

18. Which of the following approaches is the correct method for conducting the physical examination of an infant or a very young child?
    A. Toe-to-head
    B. Head-to-chest
    C. Head-to-toe
    D. Chest-to-head
    E. Both A and B

19. Poorly taken vital signs are of less value than no vital signs at all.
    A. True
    B. False

20. To obtain the blood pressure of a pediatric patient, the cuff should be _____ the width of the patient's arm.
    A. one-fourth
    B. one-third
    C. one-half
    D. two-thirds
    E. three-fourths

21. Ensure the patient is not being hyperventilated if the PETCO$_2$ is consistently
    A. 10 to 15 mmHg.
    B. less than 10 to 15 mmHg.
    C. greater than 10 to 15 mmHg.
    D. 15 to 20 mmHg.
    E. greater than 15 to 20 mmHg.

22. The hallmark of pediatric management is
    A. frequent pulse checks.
    B. prompt transport.
    C. administration of fluids.
    D. adequate oxygenation.
    E. diagnosis of medical conditions.

23. As a rule, an oropharyngeal airway should only be used on pediatric patients who
    A. have sustained head or facial trauma.
    B. are known to suffer from seizures.
    C. show signs of cardiac arrest.
    D. exhibit a vagal response.
    E. lack a gag reflex.

24. The only indication for cricothyrotomy in the pediatric patient is
    A. a foreign body airway obstruction.
    B. desire to suction the airway.
    C. failure to obtain an airway by any other method.
    D. inability to adequately ventilate by BVM.
    E. both A and C.

25. An indication for performing an endotracheal intubation in a pediatric patient is the
    A. need to gain access for deep suctioning.
    B. necessity of providing a route for drug administration.
    C. need for prolonged artificial ventilations.
    D. failure to provide adequate ventilations with a BVM.
    E. all of the above.

26. The optimal positioning of the head for pediatric intubation in the absence of a spinal injury is
    A. neutral.   D. head-tilt.
    B. hyperextended.   E. spine.
    C. sniffing.

27. If gastric distention is present in a pediatric patient, a paramedic might consider placing a(n)
    A. oropharyngeal airway.   D. nasogastric tube.
    B. nasopharyngeal airway.   E. endotracheal tube.
    C. needle cricothyrotomy.

28. In obtaining vascular access in a pediatric patient, the external jugular vein should only be used in life-threatening situations.
    A. True
    B. False

29. The indications for use of intraosseous infusion include all of the following, EXCEPT
    A. for large volumes of fluids.
    B. for existence of shock or cardiac arrest.
    C. for presence of a fracture in the pelvis.
    D. for an unresponsive patient.
    E. for failure to place a peripheral IV.

30. You are more likely to use electrical therapy on pediatric patients than on adult patients.
    A. True
    B. False

31. All of the following are symptoms of epiglottitis, EXCEPT
    A. a rapid onset.
    B. inspiratory stridor.
    C. a barking cough.
    D. drooling.
    E. a fever of approximately 102 to 104°F.

32. In treating a patient with epiglottitis, a paramedic should
    A. take the blood pressure regularly.
    B. attempt to visualize the oropharynx.
    C. take the child's temperature orally.
    D. place the child in a supine position.
    E. none of the above.

33. Common causes of lower airway distress include all of the following, EXCEPT
    A. pneumonia.   D. bronchiolitis.
    B. asthma.   E. status asthmaticus.
    C. croup.

34. When a child experiences a severe asthma attack without wheezing, this is
   A. an ominous sign.
   B. because of a lack of expectorant.
   C. a sign of improvement.
   D. because of an inability to cough.
   E. common, and should not alarm the paramedic.

35. All of the following are signs and symptoms of shock in a child, EXCEPT
   A. pale, cool, clammy skin.
   B. impaired mental status.
   C. absence of tears when crying.
   D. increased urination.
   E. a rapid respiratory rate.

36. Cardiogenic shock is more frequently encountered in prehospital pediatric care than noncardiogenic shock.
   A. True
   B. False

37. When arrhythmias do occur in children, the most common form is a(n)
   A. bradydysrhythmia.
   B. supraventricular tachydysrhythmia.
   C. ventricular tachydysrhythmia.
   D. asystole.
   E. ventricular fibrillation.

38. A pediatric patient is seen by a paramedic for a seizure. Assessment and history reveal that the child has a fever of 101°F, was very sleepy and irritable before the seizure, and has had no similar episodes. The child complained of a stiff neck and headache earlier in the day. You suspect that the episode may have been caused by
   A. febrile convulsions.
   B. meningitis.
   C. hypoglycemia.
   D. hypoxia.
   E. hyperglycemia.

39. Whenever a glucometer reading reveals a blood sugar of less than 70 mg/dL, a paramedic might suspect
   A. hypoxia.
   B. hyperglycemia.
   C. hypoglycemia.
   D. ketoacidosis.
   E. dehydration.

40. The single most common cause of trauma-related injuries in children is
   A. motor vehicle collisions.
   B. burns.
   C. falls.
   D. physical abuse.
   E. drownings.

41. Appropriate-sized pediatric immobilization equipment includes all of the following, EXCEPT
   A. towel or blanket roll.
   B. vest-type device (KED).
   C. sandbag.
   D. straps and cravats.
   E. padding.

42. All of the following are true statements about SIDS, EXCEPT that it
   A. occurs most frequently in the fall and winter.
   B. is not caused by external suffocation by blankets.
   C. tends to be more common in females than in males.
   D. is not thought to be hereditary.
   E. is possibly linked to a prone sleeping position.

43. Child abuse can take the form of
   A. psychological abuse.
   B. physical abuse.
   C. sexual abuse.
   D. neglect.
   E. all of the above.

©2013 Pearson Education, Inc.
Paramedic Care: Principles & Practice, Vol. 6, 4th Ed.

_____ **44.** In cases of suspected child abuse, management goals include all of the following, EXCEPT
   A. protection of the child from further injury.
   B. notification of proper authorities.
   C. appropriate treatment of injuries.
   D. cross-examination of the parents or caregivers.
   E. documentation of all findings and statements.

_____ **45.** A surgical connection that runs from the brain to the abdomen in a pediatric patient is called a(n)
   A. central IV.   **D.** inner cannula.
   B. tracheostomy.   **E.** epigastric tube.
   C. shunt.

MATCHING

Write the letter of the term in the space provided next to the appropriate description.

   A. greenstick fracture

   B. hypoglycemia

   C. bronchiolitis

   D. hyperglycemia

   E. epiglottitis

   F. febrile seizures

   G. tracheostomy

   H. cardiogenic shock

   I. bacterial tracheitis

   J. croup

   K. buckle fracture

   L. neonate

   M. stoma

   N. distributive shock

   O. status epilepticus

   P. bend fractures

   Q. GCS

   R. EMSC

   S. congenital

   T. growth plate

_____ **46.** Surgical incision in the neck held open by a metal or plastic tube

_____ **47.** Permanent surgical opening in the neck through which the patient breathes

_____ **48.** Scoring system for monitoring the neurological status of a patient with a possible head injury

_____ **49.** Fracture characterized by angulation and deformity in the bone without an obvious break

_____ **50.** Fracture characterized by a raised or bulging projection at the fracture site

_____ **51.** Fractures characterized by an incomplete break in the bone

_____ **52.** Abnormally high concentration of glucose in the blood

_____ **53.** Laryngotracheobronchitis; common viral infection of young children

_____ **54.** Abnormally low concentration of glucose in the blood

_____ **55.** Seizures that occur as a result of a sudden increase in temperature

_____ **56.** Prolonged seizure or multiple seizures with no regaining of consciousness between them

_____ **57.** Marked decrease in peripheral vascular resistance and consequent hypertension

_____ **58.** Inability of the heart to meet the metabolic needs of the body, resulting in inadequate tissue perfusion

_____ **59.** Viral infection of the medium-sized airways, occurring most frequently during the first year of life

_____ **60.** Bacterial infection of the airway, subglottic region

_____ **61.** Bacterial infection of the epiglottis, usually occurring in children older than age 4

_____ **62.** Area in a long bone in which growth in bone length occurs

_____ **63.** Federally funded program aimed at improving the health of pediatric patients who suffer from life-threatening illnesses and injuries

_____ **64.** Child less than 1 month old

_____ **65.** Present at birth

Special Project

Burn Injuries

Burn injuries are the leading cause of accidental death in the home for children under 14 years of age. As with other assessment tools, you must modify the "rule of nines" to estimate the extent of a burn in a pediatric patient. Read the following short patient description and complete the following diagram. Then answer the questions that follow.

You have been called to the scene of a fire at a single-family residence. The dispatcher tells you that a 2-year-old female patient has been critically burned. Upon arrival at the scene, first responders with the fire department lead you to the little girl. They report that the patient has full-thickness burns on the entire right arm, entire right leg, and the anterior trunk.

©2013 Pearson Education, Inc.
Paramedic Care: Principles & Practice, Vol. 6, 4th Ed.

THE RULE OF NINES

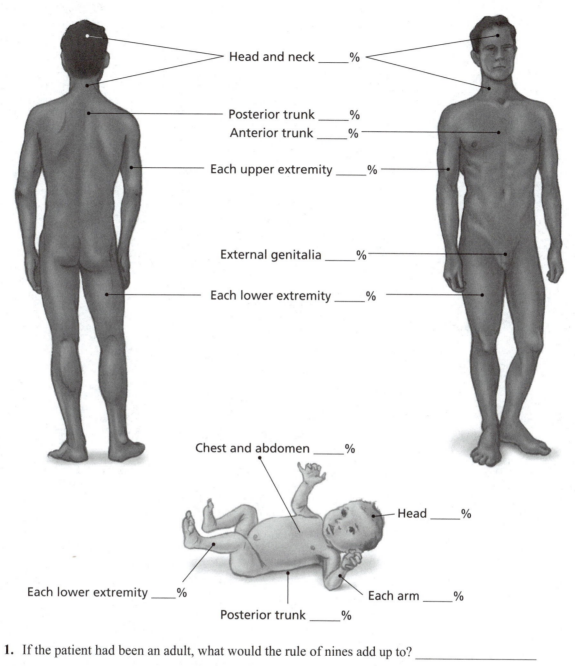

Head and neck _____%

Posterior trunk _____%
Anterior trunk _____%

Each upper extremity _____%

External genitalia _____%

Each lower extremity _____%

Chest and abdomen _____%

Head _____%

Each lower extremity _____%

Posterior trunk _____%

Each arm _____%

1. If the patient had been an adult, what would the rule of nines add up to? _____

2. What does the rule of nines add up to for this toddler? _____

3. Why do the percentages differ? _____

4. Suppose the burns had been less extensive. What alternative method for calculating the burn area might have been used? _____

Geriatrics

Review of Chapter Objectives

In each chapter of the workbook, we identify the objectives and the important elements of the text content. You should review these items and refer to the pages listed if any points are not clear.

After reading this chapter, you should be able to:

1. Define key terms introduced in this chapter.   **p. 138**

Knowing and being able to apply the key terms in each chapter is critical to understanding chapter concepts. Write the list of key terms. Then write the definition of each one in your own words. Check your understanding by confirming the definitions in the text glossary. Correct any misunderstandings. Create a study aid by writing each key term on the front of an index card and the definition on the back. Use the cards to quiz yourself, or to have someone quiz you.

2. Describe the epidemiology and demographics of aging.   **pp. 140–142**

The twentieth century, with its tremendous medical and technological advances, witnessed both a reduction in infant mortality rates and an increase in life expectancies. The cumulative effect was a population boom worldwide, with the greatest gains seen among people age 65 or older. America is getting older. Reasons for this trend include the following: the mean survival rate of older persons is increasing, the birth rate is declining, there has been an absence of major wars and other catastrophes, and health care and standards of living have improved significantly since World War II. In 2030, when the post–World War II baby boomers enter their 80s, more than 70 million people will be age 65 or older. By 2040, the elderly will represent roughly 20 percent of the population.

After years of working and/or raising a family, an elderly person must not only find new roles to fulfill but, in many cases, must also overcome the societal label of "old person." Many elderly people disprove ageism, and all the stereotypes it engenders, by living happy, productive, and active lives. Others, however, feel a sense of social isolation or uselessness. Physical and financial difficulties reinforce these feelings and help create an emotional context in which illnesses can occur.

The elderly live in both independent and dependent living environments. Many continue to live alone or with their partner well into their 80s or 90s. The "oldest" old are the most likely to live alone; in fact, nearly half of those age 85 and older live by themselves. The great majority of these people, an estimated 78 percent, are women.

Elderly persons living alone represent one of the most impoverished and vulnerable parts of society. In addition to poverty, many of the elderly who live alone, especially the old-old, have few or no living family members. Despite these difficulties, nearly 90 percent of the elderly who live alone choose to maintain their independence. Many fear any situation in which they would be treated as helpless human beings. Others do not want to burden family, friends, or even society with their problems. Some see their situation, including illness, as an inevitable part of aging and refuse to complain or ask for help. Keep this fact in mind whenever you question an elderly patient: The elderly often do not reveal problems beyond the chief complaint, either because they fear the loss of independence or because they consider the illnesses as "normal" for their age.

3. Anticipate psychosocial challenges in the elderly population.   pp. 142–144

Of the elderly people who live alone and who cannot perform some everyday tasks, nearly 74 percent receive no form of assistance. To avoid the dangers of social isolation, doctors encourage the elderly to interact with other people. This helps them to build a network of social support, a factor critical to mental health and physical well-being.

Among the elderly who receive help, more than 43 percent rely on paid assistance. Another 54 percent use unpaid assistance, and 3 percent use both types of help. Elderly people who turn to dependent care arrangements may choose among a variety of options, including live-in nursing, assisted-living facilities, life-care communities, congregate care, or personal-care homes. Approximately 5 percent of the elderly live in nursing homes.

In the course of caring for elderly patients, ethical concerns frequently arise. You may be confronted with multiple decision makers, particularly in dependent living environments. You may also have a question about the patient's competency to give informed consent or refusal of treatment. Finally, you may be faced with advance directives, such as "living wills" and do not resuscitate (DNR) orders.

Caring for an increasing number of elderly patients places a huge demand on traditional health care resources, including EMS. Currently, Social Security pays a significant portion of monthly bills, with medical support provided by four major publicly funded programs: Medicare, Medicaid, Veterans Administration (VA), and local government.

One of the biggest health care debates of the early 2000s centers around the question of preventing death at all costs. In an effort to bring down the cost of acute medical care, hospitals have shifted patient care increasingly to the home. The emphasis on home care, with appropriate medical and nursing assistance, has become a recognized medical practice. This development has gone hand-in-hand with the hospice movement, which allows terminally ill patients to live the remainder of their lives outside a hospital. Both trends impact heavily on EMS personnel, who will be called on to provide more complicated care for more patients, particularly the elderly, in an out-of-hospital setting.

4. Identify government and community resources for the elderly.   pp. 144–145

Many communities have senior centers, which provide a social atmosphere for education, recreation, and entertainment. These centers also support health care endeavors such as flu shots, blood pressure monitoring, and transport to clinics. Meals on Wheels, a program that provides from one to three meals a day, may be part of a senior volunteer organization.

Religious organizations commonly serve as a resource for the elderly. Some provide services, including dependent living environments, for their members. Others keep in touch with governmental agencies, provide food or clothing for the aged poor, and offer volunteer programs in which the elderly can make useful contributions, thus reducing their sense of isolation.

A number of associations serve as clearinghouses for information to aid the elderly. These organizations provide significant advocacy for retired persons. They often have local chapters within a county or region and usually maintain web pages, where elderly patients can access information from their homes. AARP is one of the largest, most visible, and most politically connected nonprofit organizations in the world today advocating for the elderly.

A wide range of services can be found through governmental agencies, such as the Department of Health and Human Services. Many areas maintain an office for the aging, which refers the elderly to a wide range of community programs, including nutrition centers, senior citizen law projects, home-care services, senior citizen discount programs, and transportation services.

Familiarize yourself with agencies and organizations in your area that work with the elderly. They can be found through use of the Internet, the Department of Health, or special pages in the telephone book, usually at the front or in the Yellow Pages under the heading "Senior Citizens." You can either pass this information on to elderly patients, as needed, or work with one of these groups to initiate programs such as free blood pressure checks. You might also start a prevention program that helps the elderly to safeguard their environment against fires, theft, carbon monoxide poisoning, or extremes in temperature.

©2013 Pearson Education, Inc.
Paramedic Care: Principles & Practice, Vol. 6, 4th Ed.

5. **Anticipate complex interactions between the effects of aging on the body systems and multiple disease processes in elderly patients.** pp. 145–146

In treating elderly patients, it is important to recall several facts. First, medical disorders in the elderly often present as functional impairment and should be treated as an early warning of a possibly undetected medical problem. Second, signs and symptoms do not necessarily point to the underlying cause of the problem or illness. A thorough evaluation must always be done to detect possible causes of an impairment. If identified early, an environmental- or disease-generated impairment can often be reversed. Your success depends on your knowledge of age-related changes and the implications of these changes for patient assessment and management.

Patients become less like one another as they enter their elderly years. Even so, certain generalizations can be made about age-related changes and the disease process in the elderly.

There is no escaping the fact that the body becomes less efficient with age, increasing the likelihood of malfunction. The body is susceptible to all the disorders of young people, but its maintenance, defense, and repair processes are weaker. As a result, the elderly often suffer from more than one illness or disease at a time. On average, six medical disorders may coexist in an elderly person, and perhaps even more in the old-old. Neither the patient nor the patient's doctor may be aware of all these problems. Furthermore, disease in one organ system may result in the deterioration of other systems, compounding existing acute and/or chronic conditions.

Because of concomitant diseases (comorbidity) in the elderly, complaints may not be specific to any one disorder. Common complaints of the elderly include fatigue and weakness, dizziness/vertigo/syncope, falls, headaches, insomnia, dysphagia, loss of appetite, inability to void, and constipation/diarrhea.

Elderly patients often accept medical problems as a part of aging and fail to monitor changes in their condition. In some cases, such as a silent myocardial infarction, pain may be diminished or absent. In others, an important complaint, such as constipation, may seem trivial.

Although many medical problems in the young and middle-aged populations present with a standard set of signs and symptoms, the changes involved in aging lead to different presentations. In pneumonia, for example, the classic symptom of fever is often absent in the elderly. Chest pain and a cough are also less common. Finally, many cases of pneumonia among the elderly are caused by aspiration, not infection.

6. **Explain the special considerations that necessitate maintaining a high index of suspicion for toxicologic emergencies in the elderly, including specific classes of medications that commonly result in toxicity.** pp. 146; 171–175

The existence of multiple chronic diseases in the elderly leads to the use of multiple medications. Persons age 65 and older use one-third of all prescription drugs in the United States, taking an average of 4.5 medications per day. This does not include over-the-counter (OTC) medications, vitamin supplements, or herbal remedies.

If medications are not correctly monitored, polypharmacy can lead to a number of problems among the elderly. In general, a person's sensitivity to drugs increases with age. When compared with younger patients, the elderly experience more adverse drug reactions, more drug–drug interactions, and more drug–disease interactions. Because of age-related pharmacokinetic changes such as a loss of body fluid and atrophy of organs, drugs concentrate more readily in the plasma and tissues of elderly patients. As a result, drug dosages often must be adjusted to prevent toxicity.

Aging alters pharmacokinetics and pharmacodynamics in the elderly. Functional changes in the kidneys, liver, and gastrointestinal system slow the absorption and elimination of many medications. In addition, the various compensatory mechanisms that help buffer against medication side effects are less effective in the elderly than in younger patients.

Approximately 30 percent of all hospital admissions are a result of drug-related illnesses. About 50 percent of all drug-related deaths occur in people over age 60. Accidental overdoses may occur more frequently in the aged as a result of confusion, vision impairment, self-selection of medications, forgetfulness, and concurrent drug use. Intentional drug overdose also occurs in attempts at self-destruction.

Another complicating factor is the abuse of alcohol among the elderly. Drugs or substances that have been identified as commonly causing toxicity in the elderly include beta-blockers, antihypertensives, diuretics, angiotensin-converting enzyme (ACE) inhibitors, digitalis, antipsychotics, antidepressants, medications for Parkinson's disease, antiseizure medications, analgesics, anti-inflammatory agents, corticosteroids, and others.

7. Describe special considerations for the elderly patient regarding mobility and falls, communication difficulties, and continence and elimination. pp. 146–149

Regular exercise and a good diet are two of the most effective preventive measures for ensuring mobility among the elderly. However, not all elderly people take these measures. They may suffer from severe medical problems. They may fear for their personal safety, either from accidental injury or intentional injury. Certain medications also may increase their lethargy. Whatever the cause, a lack of mobility can have detrimental physical and emotional effects. Some of these include poor nutrition, difficulty with elimination, poor skin integrity, a greater predisposition for falls, loss of independence and/or confidence, depression from "feeling old," and isolation and lack of a social network.

Fall-related injuries represent the leading cause of accidental death among the elderly and the seventh highest cause of death overall. Falls may be either intrinsic (related to the patient) or extrinsic (related to the environment). In assessing an elderly patient who has fallen, remember that a fall can result from any of multiple causes. An overmedicated patient, for example, may trip over a throw rug. A fall may also be a presenting sign of an acute illness, such as a myocardial infarction, or a sign that a chronic illness has worsened. Bear in mind the possibility of physical abuse, especially if the injury does not match the story.

Most elderly patients suffer from some form of age-related sensory changes. Normal physiologic changes may include impaired vision or blindness, impaired or loss of hearing, an altered sense of taste or smell, and/or a lower sensitivity to pain (touch). Any of these conditions can affect your ability to communicate with the patient.

The elderly often find it embarrassing to talk about problems with continence and elimination. They may feel stigmatized, isolated, and/or helpless. When confronted with these problems, do not make a big deal out of them. Respect the patient's dignity and assure the person that, in many cases, the problem is treatable. Incontinence may be either urinary or fecal. Incontinence can lead to a variety of conditions, such as rashes, skin infections, skin breakdown (ulcers), urinary tract infections, sepsis, and falls or fractures. The condition can also take a high emotional toll on both the patient and the caregiver. Difficulty with elimination can be a sign of a serious underlying condition. It can also lead to other complications. Straining to eliminate may have serious effects on the cerebral, coronary, and peripheral arterial circulations. In elderly people with cerebrovascular disease or impaired baroreceptor reflexes, efforts to force a bowel movement can lead to a transient ischemic attack (TIA) or syncope. In the case of prolonged constipation, the elderly may experience colonic ulceration, intestinal obstruction, and urinary retention.

8. Describe the importance of performing a general health assessment when caring for elderly patients. p. 149

When performing a general health assessment, take into account the patient's living situation, level of activity, network of social support, level of independence, medication history (both prescription and nonprescription), and sleep patterns. Factors in forming a general assessment include living situation, level of activity, network of social support, level of independence, medication history, and sleep patterns.

As with any person, nutrition greatly affects a patient's overall health. Patients may suffer from a number of effects of malnutrition, including vitamin deficiencies, dehydration, and hypoglycemia. Also remember that when a malnourished elderly person is fed, the food may produce other side effects, including electrolyte abnormalities, hyperglycemia, aspiration pneumonia, and a significant drop in blood pressure.

9. Adapt the scene size-up, primary assessment, patient history, secondary assessment, and use of monitoring technology to meet the needs of geriatric patients. pp. 149–152

The chief complaint of the elderly patient may seem trivial or vague at first. Also, the patient may fail to report important symptoms. Therefore, you should try to distinguish the patient's chief complaint from the patient's primary problem.

©2013 Pearson Education, Inc.
Paramedic Care: Principles & Practice, Vol. 6, 4th Ed.

The presence of multiple diseases also complicates the assessment process. The presence of chronic problems may make it more difficult to assess an acute problem. It is easy to confuse symptoms from a chronic illness with those of an acute condition. Because of the complexity of factors that can affect assessment, you must probe for significant symptoms and, ultimately, the primary problem. Patience, respect, and kindness will elicit the answers needed for a pertinent medical history.

When gathering the history, keep in mind the complications that arise from multiple diseases and multiple medications. Medications can be an especially important indicator of the patient's diseases. Therefore, you should find the patient's medications and take them to the hospital with the patient. Try to determine which of the medications, including OTC medications, are currently being taken. In cases of multiple medications, there is an increased incidence of medication errors, drug interactions, and noncompliance. Communication challenges may include visual, hearing, and/or speech impairments.

Remember that age sometimes diminishes mental status. When confronted with a confused patient, try to determine whether the patient's mental status represents a significant change from normal. Do not assume that a confused, disoriented patient is "just senile," thus failing to assess for a serious underlying problem. Another complication results from depression, which can be mistaken for many other disorders. It can often mimic senility and organic brain syndrome. Depression may also inhibit patient cooperation.

After obtaining the history, and if time allows, try to verify the patient's history with a credible source. This will often be less offensive to the patient if done out of his presence. While at the scene, it is important to observe the surroundings for indications of the patient's self-sufficiency. Look for evidence of drug or alcohol ingestion and for Medic Alert tags, Vial-of-Life, or similar medical identification items. It is also important to spot signs of abuse or neglect, particularly in dependent living arrangements.

Certain considerations must be kept in mind when examining the elderly patient. Remember that some patients may be easily fatigued and unable to tolerate a long examination. Also, because of the problems with temperature regulation, the patient may be wearing several layers of clothing, which can make examination difficult. Be sure to explain all actions clearly before initiating the examination, especially to patients with impaired vision. Be aware that the patient may minimize or deny symptoms because of a fear of becoming institutionalized or a loss of self-sufficiency.

Try to distinguish signs of chronic disease from an acute problem. Peripheral pulses may be difficult to evaluate, because of peripheral vascular disease and arthritis. The elderly may also have non-pathological crackles (rales) upon lung auscultation. In addition, the elderly often exhibit an increase in mouth breathing and a loss of skin elasticity, which may be easily confused with dehydration. Dependent edema may be caused by inactivity, not congestive heart failure. Only experience and practice will allow you to distinguish acute from chronic physical findings.

10. Anticipate common medical problems in the elderly.

In general, the elderly suffer from the same kinds of medical emergencies as younger patients. However, illnesses may be more severe, complications more likely, and classic signs and symptoms absent or altered. In addition, the elderly are more likely to react adversely to stress and deteriorate much more quickly than young or middle-aged adults. The following are some of the medical disorders that you may encounter.

Pulmonary/Respiratory Disorders   pp. 157–160

Respiratory emergencies are some of the most common reasons elderly persons summon EMS or seek emergency care.

Pneumonia. Pneumonia is an infection of the lung. It is usually caused by a bacterium or virus. However, aspiration pneumonia may also develop as a result of difficulty swallowing. Pneumonia is a serious disease for the elderly. It is the fourth-leading cause of death in people age 65 and older. Its incidence increases with age at a rate of 10 percent for each decade beyond age 20. It is found in up to 60 percent of the autopsies performed on the elderly. Reasons the elderly develop pneumonia more frequently than younger patients include decreased immune response, reduced pulmonary function, increased colonization of the pharynx by gram-negative bacteria, abnormal or ineffective cough reflex, and decreased effectiveness of mucociliary cells of the upper respiratory system.

The elderly who are at greatest risk for contracting pneumonia include frail adults and those with chronic, multiple diseases or compromised immunity. Institutionalized patients in hospitals or nursing homes are especially vulnerable because of increased exposure to microorganisms and limited mobility. A patient in an institutional setting is up to 50 times more likely to contract pneumonia than an elderly patient receiving home care.

Chronic Obstructive Pulmonary Disease. Chronic obstructive pulmonary disease (COPD) is really a collection of diseases, characterized by chronic airflow obstruction with reversible and/or irreversible components. Although each COPD has its own distinct features, elderly patients commonly have two or more types at the same time. COPD usually refers to some combination of emphysema, chronic bronchitis, and, to a lesser degree, asthma. Pneumonia, as well as other respiratory disorders, can further complicate chronic obstructive pulmonary disease in the elderly.

In the United States, chronic obstructive pulmonary disease is among the 10 leading causes of death. Its prevalence has been increasing during the past 20 years. Several factors combine to produce the damage of COPD, including genetic disposition, exposure to environmental pollutants, existence of a childhood respiratory disease, and cigarette smoking, a contributing factor in up to 80 percent of all cases of COPD.

The physiology of COPD varies, but may include inflammation of the air passages with increased mucus production or actual destruction of the alveoli. The outcome is decreased airflow in the alveoli, resulting in reduced oxygen exchange.

Pulmonary Embolism. Pulmonary embolism (PE) should always be considered as a possible cause of respiratory distress in the elderly. Although statistics for the elderly are unavailable, approximately 650,000 cases occur annually in the United States alone. Of this number, a pulmonary embolism is the primary cause of death in 100,000 people and a contributing factor in another 100,000 deaths. Nearly 11 percent of PE deaths take place in the first hour after onset and 38 percent in the second hour.

Blood clots are the most frequent cause of pulmonary embolism. However, the condition may also be caused by fat, air, bone marrow, tumor cells, or foreign bodies. Risk factors for developing pulmonary embolism include deep venous thrombosis; prolonged immobility, common among the elderly; malignancy (tumors); paralysis; fractures of the pelvis, hip, or leg; obesity; trauma to the leg vessels; major surgery; presence of a venous catheter; use of estrogen (in women); and atrial fibrillation.

Pulmonary Edema. Pulmonary edema is an effusion or escape of serous fluids into the alveoli and interstitial tissues of the lungs. Acute pulmonary edema can develop rapidly in the elderly. Although most commonly associated with acute myocardial infarction, it can also result from pulmonary infections, inhaled toxins, narcotic overdose, pulmonary embolism, and decreased atmospheric pressure.

Lung Cancer. North America has the highest incidence of lung cancer in the world. The incidence increases with age, with about 65 percent of all lung cancer deaths occurring among people age 65 and older. The leading cause of lung cancer is cigarette smoking. Often, progressive dyspnea will be the first presentation of a cancerous lesion. Hemoptysis (bloody sputum), chronic cough, and weight loss are also common symptoms.

Cardiovascular Disorders
pp. 160–162

The leading cause of death in the elderly is cardiovascular disease. Assessment and treatment of cardiovascular disease in the elderly patient is often complicated by non-age-related factors and disease processes in other organ systems.

Angina Pectoris. The likelihood of developing angina increases dramatically with age. This is especially true of women, who are protected by estrogen until after menopause. Angina is usually triggered by physical activity, especially after a meal, and by exposure to very cold weather. Attacks vary in frequency, from several a day to occasional episodes separated by weeks or months.

Myocardial Infarction. A myocardial infarction (MI) involves actual death of muscle tissue owing to a partial or complete occlusion of one or more of the coronary arteries. The greatest number of patients hospitalized for acute myocardial infarction are older than 65. The elderly patient with myocardial infarction is less likely to present with classic symptoms, such as chest pain, than a younger counterpart. Atypical presentations that may be seen in the elderly include absence of pain; exercise intolerance;

©2013 Pearson Education, Inc.
Paramedic Care: Principles & Practice, Vol. 6, 4th Ed.

confusion/dizziness; syncope; dyspnea, common in patients over age 85; neck, dental, and/or epigastric pain; and fatigue/weakness.

The mortality rate associated with myocardial infarction and/or resulting complications doubles after age 70. Unlike younger patients, the elderly are more likely to suffer a silent myocardial infarction. They also tend to have larger myocardial infarctions. The majority of deaths that occur in the first few hours following a myocardial infarction are caused by arrhythmias.

Heart Failure. Heart failure takes place when cardiac output cannot meet the body's metabolic demands. The incidence rises exponentially after age 60. The condition is widespread among the elderly and is the most common diagnosis in hospitalized patients over age 65. The causes of heart failure fall into one of four categories: impairment to flow, inadequate cardiac filling, volume overload, and myocardial failure.

Typical age-related factors, such as prolonged myocardial contractions, make the elderly vulnerable to heart failure. Other factors that place them at risk include noncompliance with drug therapy, anemia, ischemia, thermoregulatory disorders (hypothermia/hyperthermia), hypoxia, infection, use of nonsteroidal anti-inflammatory drugs, and arrhythmias.

Arrhythmias. Many cardiac arrhythmias develop with age. Atrial fibrillation is the most common arrhythmia encountered and can be a predictor of long-term mortality in elderly patients. Arrhythmias occur primarily as a result of degeneration of the patient's conductive system. Anything that decreases myocardial blood flow can produce an arrhythmia. They may also be caused by electrolyte abnormalities.

To complicate matters further, the elderly do not tolerate extremes in heart rate as well as a younger person would. For example, a heart rate of 140 in an older patient may cause syncope, whereas a younger patient can often tolerate a heart rate greater than 180. In addition, arrhythmias can lead to falls from cerebral hypoperfusion. They can also result in congestive heart failure (CHF) or a transient ischemic attack.

Aortic Dissection/Aneurysms. Aortic dissection is a degeneration of the wall of the aorta, either in the thoracic or abdominal cavity. It can result in an aneurysm or in a rupture of the vessel. Approximately 80 percent of thoracic aneurysms are the result of atherosclerosis combined with hypertension. The remaining cases occur secondary to other factors, including Marfan syndrome or blunt trauma to the chest. Patients with dissections will often present with tearing chest pain radiating through to the back or, if rupture occurs, cardiac arrest. The distal portion of the aorta is the most common site for abdominal aneurysms. Approximately 1 in 250 people over age 50 die from a ruptured abdominal aneurysm.

Hypertension. Hypertension appears to be a product of industrial society. In developed nations, such as the United States, the systolic and diastolic pressures have a tendency to rise until age 60. Systolic pressure may continue to rise after that time, but diastolic pressure stabilizes. Because this rise in blood pressure is not seen in less developed nations, experts believe that hypertension is not a normal age-related change.

Today more than 50 percent of Americans over age 65 have clinically diagnosed hypertension, which is defined as blood pressure greater than 140/90 mmHg. Prolonged elevated blood pressure will eventually damage the heart, brain, and/or kidneys. As a result of hypertension, elderly patients are at greater risk for heart failure, stroke, blindness, renal failure, coronary heart disease, and peripheral vascular disease. In men with blood pressure greater than 160/95 mmHg, the risk of mortality nearly doubles.

Hypertension increases with atherosclerosis, which is more common with the elderly than other age groups. Other contributing factors include obesity and diabetes. The condition can be prevented or controlled through diet (sodium reduction), exercise, cessation of smoking, and compliance with medications.

Syncope. Syncope is a common presenting complaint among the elderly. The condition results when blood flow to the brain is temporarily interrupted or decreased. It is most often caused by problems with either the nervous system or the cardiovascular system. In general, syncope has a higher incidence of death in elderly patients than in younger individuals. Some of the common presentations that you may encounter include vasodepressor syncope, orthostatic syncope, vasovagal syncope, cardiac syncope, seizures, and transient ischemic attacks.

Elderly patients are at risk for several neurologic emergencies. Often, the exact cause is not initially known and may require probing at the hospital. Many of the neurologic disorders that you will encounter in the field will exhibit an alteration in mental status. You may discover a range of underlying causes from stroke to degenerative brain disease. Some of the most common causes of altered mental status include cerebrovascular disease (stroke or transient ischemic attack), myocardial infarction, seizures, medication-related problems (drug interactions, drug underdose, and drug overdose), infection, fluid and electrolyte abnormalities (dehydration), lack of nutrients (hypoglycemia), temperature changes (hypothermia, hyperthermia), and structural changes (dementia, subdural hematoma).

Cerebrovascular Disease (Stroke/TIAs). Stroke is a leading cause of death in the United States. Annually, about 500,000 people suffer strokes and about 150,000 die. Incidence of stroke and the likelihood of dying from a stroke increase with age. Occlusive stroke is statistically more common in the elderly and relatively uncommon in younger individuals. Older patients are at higher risk of stroke because of atherosclerosis, hypertension, immobility, limb paralysis, congestive heart failure, and atrial fibrillation.

Transient ischemic attacks are also more common in older patients. More than one-third of patients suffering TIAs will develop a major, permanent stroke. As previously mentioned, TIAs are a frequent cause of syncope in the elderly.

Strokes usually fall into one of two major categories. Brain ischemia—injury to brain tissue caused by an inadequate supply of oxygen and nutrients—accounts for about 80 percent of all strokes. Brain hemorrhage, the second major category, may be either subarachnoid hemorrhage or intracerebral hemorrhage. These different patterns of bleeding have different presentations, causes, and treatments. However, together they account for a high percentage of all stroke deaths.

Seizures. Seizures can be easily mistaken for strokes in the elderly. In addition, a first-time seizure may occur as a result of damage from a previous stroke. Not all seizures experienced by the elderly are of the major motor type. Some are more subtle. Many causes of seizure activity in the elderly have been identified. Common causes include seizure disorder (epilepsy), syncope, recent or past head trauma, mass lesion (tumor or bleed), alcohol withdrawal, hypoglycemia, and stroke.

Dizziness/Vertigo. Dizziness is a frightening experience and a frequent complaint of the elderly. The complaint of dizziness may actually mean that the patient has suffered syncope, presyncope, lightheadedness, or true vertigo. Vertigo is a specific sensation of motion perceived by the patient as spinning or whirling. Many patients will report that they feel as though they are spinning. Vertigo is often accompanied by sweating, pallor, nausea, and vomiting. Meniere's disease can cause severe, intractable vertigo. It is often, however, associated with a constant "roaring" sound in the ears, as well as ear "pressure."

Delirium. Approximately 15 percent of all Americans over age 65 have some degree of dementia or delirium. Delirium is a global mental impairment of sudden onset and self-limited duration. Many conditions can cause delirium. The cause may be either organic brain disease or disorders that occur elsewhere in the body. Delirium in the elderly is a serious condition. According to some estimates, about 18 percent of hospitalized elderly patients with delirium die. Possible etiologies or causes include subdural hematoma, tumors and other mass lesions, drug-induced changes or alcohol intoxication, CNS infections, electrolyte abnormalities, heart failure, fever, metabolic disorders, including hypoglycemia, chronic endocrine abnormalities (including hypothyroidism and hyperthyroidism), and postconcussion syndrome.

Dementia. Approximately 15 percent of all Americans over age 65 have some degree of dementia or delirium. Dementia is a chronic global cognitive impairment, often progressive or irreversible. Dementia is more prevalent in the elderly than delirium. More than 50 percent of all nursing home patients have some form of dementia. It is usually caused by an underlying neurologic disease. This mental deterioration is often called "organic brain syndrome," "senile dementia," or "senility." It is important to find out whether an alteration in mental status is acute or chronic. Causes of dementia include small strokes, atherosclerosis, age-related neurologic changes, neurologic diseases, certain hereditary diseases, and Alzheimer's disease.

©2013 Pearson Education, Inc.
Paramedic Care: Principles & Practice, Vol. 6, 4th Ed.

Alzheimer's Disease. The best known form of dementia is Alzheimer's disease, a condition that affects 5.5 million Americans. Alzheimer's disease, a particular type of dementia, is a chronic degenerative disorder that attacks the brain and results in impaired memory, thinking, and behavior. It accounts for more than half of all forms of dementia in the elderly.

Parkinson's Disease. Parkinson's disease is a degenerative disorder characterized by changes in muscle response, including tremors, loss of facial expression, and gait disturbances. It mainly appears in people over age 50 and peaks at age 70. The disease affects about 1 million Americans, with 50,000 new cases diagnosed each year. It is the fourth most common neurodegenerative disease among the elderly.

The cause of primary Parkinson's disease remains unknown. However, it affects the basal ganglia in the brain, an area that deciphers messages going to muscles. Secondary Parkinson's disease is distinguished from primary Parkinson's disease by having a known cause. Some of the most common causes include viral encephalitis, atherosclerosis of cerebral vessels, reaction to certain drugs or toxins, metabolic disorders such as anoxia, tumors, head trauma, and degenerative disorders such as Shy-Drager syndrome.

Metabolic and Endocrine Disorders   pp. 165–166

The endocrine system undergoes a number of age-related changes that affect hormone levels. The most common endocrine disorders include diabetes mellitus and problems related to the thyroid gland. Of the two, you will more often treat diabetic-related emergencies, particularly hypoglycemia.

Diabetes Mellitus. An estimated 20 percent of older adults have diabetes mellitus, primarily type 2 diabetes. Almost 40 percent have some type of glucose intolerance. The elderly develop these disorders for these reasons: poor diet, decreased physical activity, loss of lean body mass, impaired insulin production, and resistance by body cells to the actions of insulin.

Diagnosis of type 2 diabetes usually occurs during routine screening in a physical exam. In some cases, urine tests may register negative because of an increased renal glucose threshold in the elderly. The condition may present, in its early stages, with vague constitutional symptoms such as fatigue or weakness. Allowed to progress, diabetes can result in neuropathy and visual impairment. These manifestations often lead to more aggressive blood testing, which in most cases will reveal elevated glucose levels.

The treatment of diabetes involves diet, exercise, the use of sulfonylurea agents, and/or insulin. Many diabetics use self-monitoring devices to test glucose levels. Unfortunately, the cost of these devices and the accompanying test strips sometimes discourages the elderly from using them. Elderly patients on insulin also risk hypoglycemia, especially if they accidentally take too much insulin or do not eat enough food following injection. The lack of good nutrition can be particularly troublesome to elderly diabetics. They often find it difficult to prepare meals, fail to enjoy food because of altered taste perceptions, have trouble chewing food, or are unable to purchase adequate and/or the correct food because of limited income.

Thyroid Disorders. With normal aging, the thyroid gland undergoes moderate atrophy and changes in hormone production. An estimated 2 percent to 5 percent of people over age 65 experience hypothyroidism, a condition resulting from inadequate levels of thyroid hormones. It affects women in greater numbers than men, and the prevalence rises with age.

Gastrointestinal Disorders   pp. 166–167

Gastrointestinal (GI) emergencies are common among the elderly. The most frequent emergency is gastrointestinal bleeding. However, older people will also describe a variety of other gastrointestinal complaints: nausea, poor appetite, diarrhea, and constipation, to name a few. Remember that, like other presenting complaints, these conditions may be symptomatic of more serious diseases. Bowel problems, for example, may point to cancer of the colon or other abdominal organs.

Some of the most critical GI problems that you may encounter in the field will involve internal hemorrhage and bowel obstruction. You may also be called upon to treat mesenteric ischemia or infarct, a serious and life-threatening condition in an elderly patient.

GI Hemorrhage. Gastrointestinal bleeding falls into two general categories: upper GI bleed and lower GI bleed. Upper gastrointestinal bleeding includes peptic ulcer disease, gastritis, esophageal varices, and Mallory-Weiss tear. Lower gastrointestinal bleeding includes diverticulosis, tumors, ischemic colitis, and arterio-venous malformations.

Bowel Obstruction. Bowel obstruction in the elderly typically involves the small bowel. Causes include tumors, prior abdominal surgery, use of certain medications, and occasionally the presence of vertebral compression fractures.

Mesenteric Ischemia/Infarct. Vessels arising from the superior or inferior mesenteric arteries generally serve the bowel. An infarct occurs when a portion of the bowel does not receive enough blood to survive. Certain age-related changes make the elderly more vulnerable to this condition. First, as a person ages, changes in the heart (such as atrial fibrillation) or the vessels (atherosclerosis) predispose the patient to a clot lodging in one of the branches serving the bowel. Second, changes in the bowel itself can promote swelling that effectively cuts off blood flow.

Skin Disorders   pp. 167–168

Younger and older adults experience common skin disorders at about the same rates. However, age-related changes in the immune system make the elderly more prone to certain chronic skin diseases and infections. They are also more likely to develop pressure ulcers (bedsores) than any other age group.

Skin Diseases. Elderly patients commonly complain about pruritus, or itching. This condition can be caused by dermatitis (eczema) or environmental conditions, especially during winter (i.e., from hot dry air in the home and cold windy air outside). Keep in mind that generalized itching can also be a sign of systemic diseases, particularly liver and renal disorders. When itching is strong and unrelenting, suspect an underlying disease and encourage the patient to seek medical evaluation.

Slower healing and compromised tissue perfusion in the elderly make them more susceptible to bacterial infection of wounds, appearing as cellulitis, impetigo, and, in the case of immunocompromised adults, staphylococcal scalded skin. The elderly also experience a higher incidence of fungal infections, partly because of decreases in the cutaneous immunologic response. In addition, they suffer higher rates of herpes zoster (shingles), which peaks between ages 50 and 70. Although these skin disorders also occur in the young, their duration and severity increases markedly with age.

Pressure Ulcers (Decubitus Ulcers). Most pressure ulcers occur in people over age 70. As many as 20 percent of patients enter the hospital with a pressure ulcer or develop one while hospitalized. The highest incidence occurs in nursing homes, where up to 25 percent of patients may develop this condition.

Pressure ulcers typically develop from the waist down, usually over bony prominences, in bedridden patients. However, they can occur anywhere on the body and with the patient in any position. Pressure ulcers usually result from tissue hypoxia and affect the skin, subcutaneous tissues, and muscle. Factors that can increase the risk of this condition include external compression of tissues, altered sensory perception, maceration caused by excessive moisture, decreased activity, decreased mobility, poor nutrition, and friction or shear.

Musculoskeletal Disorders   pp. 168–170

The skeleton, as you know, is a metabolically active organ. Its metabolic processes are influenced by a number of factors, including age, diet, exercise, and hormone levels. The musculoskeletal system is also subject to disease. In fact, musculoskeletal diseases are the leading cause of functional impairment in the elderly. Although usually not fatal, musculoskeletal disorders often produce chronic disability, which in turn creates a context for illness. Two of the most widespread musculoskeletal disorders include osteoarthritis and osteoporosis.

Osteoarthritis. Osteoarthritis is the leading cause of disability among people age 65 and older. Many experts think the condition may not be one disease but several with similar presentations. Although wear and tear, as well as age-related changes such as loss of muscle mass, predispose the elderly to osteoarthritis, other factors may play a role as well. Presumed contributing causes include: obesity, primary disorders of the joint, trauma, and congenital abnormalities.

©2013 Pearson Education, Inc.
Paramedic Care: Principles & Practice, Vol. 6, 4th Ed.

Osteoporosis. Osteoporosis affects an estimated 20 million Americans and is largely responsible for fractures of the hip, wrist, and vertebral bones following a fall or other injury. Risk factors include:

- Age. Peak bone mass for men and women occurs in their third and fourth decades of life and declines at varying rates thereafter. Decreased bone density generally becomes a treatment consideration at about age 50.
- Gender. The decline of estrogen production places women at a higher risk of developing osteoporosis than men. Women are more than twice as likely to have brittle bones, especially if they experience early menopause (before age 45) and do not take estrogen replacement therapy.
- Race. Whites and Asians are more likely to develop osteoporosis than African Americans and Latinos, who have higher bone mass at skeletal peak.
- Body weight. Thin people, or people with low body weight, are at greater risk of osteoporosis than obese people. Increased skeletal weight is thought to promote bone density. However, weight-bearing exercise can have the same effect.
- Family history. Genetic factors (i.e., peak bone mass attainment) and a family history of fractures may predispose a person to osteoporosis.
- Miscellaneous. Late menarche, nulliparity, and use of caffeine, alcohol, and cigarettes are all thought to be important determinants of bone mass.

Ankylosing Spondylitis. Aankylosing spondylitis (AS) is a form of inflammatory arthritis that primarily affects the spine. It is estimated that approximately 500,000 people in the United States have the disease. AS primarily causes inflammation of the joints between the vertebrae of the spine and the sacroiliac joints in the pelvis. It can also cause inflammation and pain in other parts of the body. As the condition worsens and the inflammation persists, new bone forms as a part of the healing process. The bone may grow from the edge of the vertebra across the disk space between two vertebrae, resulting in a bony bridge; this may occur throughout the spine so that the spine becomes stiff and inflexible—effectively fusing the spine. On spinal X-rays, this phenomenon is referred to as "bamboo spine." This fusion can also affect the rib cage, restricting lung capacity and function.

As the disease progresses, the spine becomes fused into a single unit incapable of flexion, extension, or lateral movement. Usually the fusion progresses with the spine assuming a flexed position and the patient is forced to walk bent over.

Renal Disorders p. 170

The most common renal diseases in the elderly include renal failure, glomerulonephritis, and renal blood clots. These problems may be traced to two age-related factors: (1) loss in kidney size and (2) changes in the walls of the renal arteries and in the arterioles serving the glomeruli. In general, a person's kidney loses approximately one-third of its weight between the ages of 30 and 80. Most of this loss occurs in the tissues that filter blood. When filtering tissue is gone, blood is shunted from the precapillary side directly to venules on the postcapillary side, thus bypassing any tissue still capable of filtering. The result is a reduction in kidney efficiency. This condition is complicated by changes in renal arteries, which promote the development of renal emboli and thrombi.

With renal changes, elderly patients are more likely to accumulate toxins and medications within the bloodstream. Occasionally, this will be obvious to the patient because he will experience a substantial decrease in urine output. More often, however, the elderly are prone to a type of renal failure in which urine output remains normal to high while the kidney remains ineffective in clearing wastes.

Processes that precipitate acute renal failure include hypotension, heart failure, major surgery, sepsis, angiographic procedures (the dye is nephrotoxic), and use of nephrotoxic antibiotics (i.e., gentamycin, tobramycin). Ongoing hypertension also figures in the development of chronic renal failure.

Urinary Disorders p. 170

Urinary tract infections (UTIs) affect as much as 10 percent of the elderly population each year. Younger women generally suffer more UTIs than young men, but in the elderly the distribution is almost even. Most of these infections result from bacteria and easily lead to urosepsis owing to reduced immune system function among the elderly.

A number of factors contribute to the high rate of UTIs among the elderly: bladder outlet obstruction from benign prostatic hyperplasia (in men), atrophic vaginitis (in women), stroke, immobilization, use of indwelling bladder catheters, diabetes, upper urinary tract stone, and dementia, with resulting poor hygiene.

11. Describe special considerations in the elderly that necessitate maintaining a high index of suspicion for environmental emergencies. pp. 170–171

The elderly are highly susceptible to variations in environmental temperatures. This occurs in the elderly because of altered or impaired thermoregulatory mechanisms. In addition, the elderly may have a diminished perception of cold temperatures. Drugs and disease can further affect an elderly patient's response to temperature extremes, resulting in hyperthermia or accidental hypothermia. Environmental emergencies are common causes of EMS calls, especially among the elderly living alone or in poverty. Nearly 50 percent of all heatstroke deaths in the United States occur among people over age 50. The elderly are just as susceptible to low temperatures, suffering about 750,000 winter deaths annually, primarily from hypothermia and "winter risks" such as pneumonia and influenza.

A number of factors predispose the elderly to hypothermia, including accidental exposure to cold, CNS disorders, endocrine disorders, drugs that interfere with heat production, malnutrition or starvation, chronic illness, forced inactivity, low or fixed income, inflammatory dermatitis, and AV shunts.

Signs and symptoms of hypothermia can be slow to develop. Many times, elderly patients with hypothermia lose their sensitivity to cold and fail to complain. Nonspecific complaints may suggest a metabolic disorder or stroke. Hypothermic patients may exhibit slow speech, confusion, and sleepiness. In the early stages, patients will exhibit hypertension and an increased heart rate. As hypothermia progresses, however, blood pressure drops and the heart rate slows, sometimes to a barely detectable level.

Remember that the elderly patient with hypothermia often does not shiver. Check the abdomen and back to see if the skin is cool to the touch. Expect subcutaneous tissues to be firm. If your unit has a low-temperature thermometer, check the patient's core temperature. As with other medical disorders, prevention is the preferred treatment. Focus on the rewarming techniques used with other patients and rapid transport.

Age-related changes in sweat glands and increased incidence of heart disease place the elderly at risk of heat stress. They may develop heat cramps, heat exhaustion, or heatstroke. Although the first two disorders rarely result in death, heatstroke is a serious medical emergency. Risk factors for severe hyperthermia include altered sensory output, inadequate liquid intake, decreased functioning of the thermoregulatory center, commonly prescribed medications that inhibit sweating, low or fixed income, alcoholism, concomitant medical disorders, and use of diuretics.

Like hypothermia, early heatstroke may present with nonspecific signs and symptoms, such as nausea, light-headedness, dizziness, or headache. High temperature is the most reliable indicator, but consider even a slight temperature elevation as symptomatic if coupled with an absence of sweating and neurologic impairment. Severe hypotension also exists in many critical patients. Prevention strategies include adequate fluid intake, reduced activity, shelter in an air-conditioned environment, and use of light clothing. If hyperthermia develops, however, rapid treatment and transport are necessary.

12. Describe special considerations in the elderly that necessitate maintaining a high index of suspicion for behavioral and psychiatric problems, including risk of suicide. pp. 175–176

When behavioral or psychological problems develop later in life, they are often dismissed as normal age-related changes. This attitude denies an elderly person the opportunity to correct a treatable condition and/or overlooks an underlying physical disorder. Unless an organic brain disorder is involved, alterations in behavior should be considered symptomatic of a possible psychological problem.

It is important to keep in mind the emotionally stressful situations facing many elderly people: isolation, loneliness, loss of self-dependence, loss of strength, fear of the future, and more. Up to 15 percent of the noninstitutionalized elderly experience depression. Within institutions, that figure rises to about 30 percent. Depression is the leading cause of suicide among the elderly.

The highest suicide rates in the United States are among people over age 65, especially men. The elderly account for 20 percent of all suicides, but represent only 12 percent of the total population. Someone over age 65 completes suicide about every 90 minutes. Suicide is the third-leading cause of death among the elderly, following falls and car accidents.

©2013 Pearson Education, Inc.
Paramedic Care: Principles & Practice, Vol. 6, 4th Ed.

Suicidal behavior is related to stress. In cases of a seriously depressed patient, elicit behavior patterns from family, friends, or caregivers. Warning signs may include loss of interest in activities that were once enjoyable; curtailing social interaction, grooming, and self-care; breaking from medical or exercise regimens; grieving a personal loss; feeling useless; putting affairs in order; giving away things; finalizing a will; and stockpiling medications or other lethal means of self-destruction.

13. Describe special considerations in the elderly that increase the risk of particular injuries and impair the elderly patient's physiologic response to injuries. p. 176

Trauma is the leading cause of death among the elderly. Older patients who sustain moderate to severe injuries are more likely to die than their younger counterparts. Post-injury disability is also more common in the elderly than in the young. A number of factors contribute to the high incidence and severity of trauma among the elderly. Slower reflexes, arthritis, and diminished eyesight and hearing predispose the elderly to accidents, especially falls. The elderly, because of their physical state and vulnerability, are also at high risk from trauma caused by criminal assault.

Orthopedic Injuries pp. 177–178

The elderly suffer the greatest mortality and greatest incidence of disability from falls. Approximately 33 percent of the falls in the elderly result in at least one fractured bone. The most common fall-related fracture is a fracture of the hip or pelvis. Falls also result in a variety of stress fractures in the elderly, including fractures of the proximal humerus, distal radius, proximal tibia, and thoracic and lumbar bodies. In treating orthopedic injuries, remember to ask questions aimed at detecting an underlying medical condition.

Burns pp. 178–179

People age 60 and older are more likely to suffer death from burns than any other age group except neonates and infants. Factors that help explain the high mortality rate among the elderly include age-related changes that slow reaction time, preexisting diseases that increase the risk of medical complications, age-related skin changes (thinning) that increase the severity of burns, immunological and metabolic changes that increase the risk of infection, and reductions in physiologic function and the reduced reserves of several organ systems that make the elderly more vulnerable to systemic stress.

Head and Spinal Injuries p. 179

As people age, the brain decreases in size and weight. The skull, however, remains constant in size, allowing the brain more room to move, thus increasing the likelihood of brain injury. Because of this, the signs and symptoms of brain injury may develop more slowly in the elderly patient, sometimes over days or weeks. In fact, the patient may often have forgotten the offending incident.

The cervical spine is also more susceptible to injury due to osteoporosis and spondylosis—a degeneration of the vertebral body. In addition, arthritic changes can gradually compress the nerve rootlets or spinal cord. Thus, injury to the spine in the elderly makes them much more susceptible to spinal cord injury.

14. Relate the pathophysiology of specific geriatric problems to the priorities of patient assessment and management. p. 152

Each elderly patient presents a unique challenge in terms of assessment and management. You will need to tailor your management plan to fit a patient's illness, injury, and overall general health. Because of the potential for rapid deterioration among the elderly, you must quickly spot conditions requiring rapid transport.

As with any other patient, your first concern is the primary assessment. Remain alert at all times for changes in an elderly patient's neurologic status, vital signs, and general cardiac status.

In general, remember that transport to a hospital is often more stressful for the elderly than for any other age group, except for the very young. Avoid lights and sirens in all but the most serious cases, such as when you suspect a pulmonary embolism or bowel infarction. A calm, smooth transport helps to reduce patient anxiety—and the resulting strain that anxiety places on an elderly patient's heart.

Provide emotional support at every phase of the call. Nearly any serious illness or injury in the elderly can provoke a sense of impending doom. Death is a very real possibility to this age group.

Pulmonary/Respiratory Disorders

pp. 157–160

Pneumonia. Common signs and symptoms of pneumonia include increasing dyspnea, congestion, fever, chills, tachypnea, sputum production, and altered mental status. Occasionally, abdominal pain may be the only symptom. Because of thermoregulatory changes, a fever may be absent in an elderly patient.

Prevention strategies include prophylactic treatment with antibiotics. Efforts should also be taken to reduce exposure to infectious patients and to promote patient mobility. In treating an elderly patient with pneumonia, manage all life threats. Maintain adequate oxygenation. Transport the patient to the hospital for diagnosis, keeping in mind that patients with respiratory disease often have other underlying problems.

Chronic Obstructive Pulmonary Disease. Usual signs and symptoms include cough, increased sputum production, dyspnea, accessory muscle use, pursed-lip breathing, tripod positioning, exercise intolerance, wheezing, pleuritic chest pain, and tachypnea.

COPD is progressive and debilitating. The patient can often keep the signs and symptoms under control until the body is stressed. When the condition becomes disabling, it is called exacerbation of COPD. This condition can lead rapidly to patient death because the accompanying hypoxia and hypercapnia alter the acid–base balance and deprive the tissues of the oxygen needed for efficient energy production.

The most effective prevention involves elimination of tobacco products and reduced exposure to cigarette smoke (in nonsmokers). Recent legislation has sought to keep public places smoke free and to discourage cigarette smoking in the young. Once the disease is present, patients are taught to identify stresses that exacerbate the condition. Appropriate self-care includes exercise, avoidance of infections, appropriate use of drugs, and, when necessary, calling EMS.

When confronted with an elderly patient with COPD, treatment is essentially the same as for all age groups. Supply supplemental oxygen to correct hypoxia and possibly drug therapy, usually for reducing dyspnea.

Pulmonary Embolism. Pulmonary emboli usually originate in the deep veins of the thigh and calf. The condition should be suspected in any patient with the acute onset of dyspnea. Often, it is accompanied by pleuritic chest pain and right heart failure. If the pulmonary embolus is massive, you can often expect severe dyspnea, cardiac arrhythmias, and, ultimately, cardiovascular collapse.

Definitive diagnosis of a pulmonary embolism takes place in a hospital setting. The goals of field treatment are to manage and minimize complications of the condition. General treatment considerations include delivery of supplemental oxygen via mask to maintain a SpO_2 of 92 percent to 94 percent. Establishment of an IV for possible administration of medications is appropriate, but vigorous fluid therapy should be avoided, if possible.

Prehospital pharmacologic therapy for pulmonary embolism is limited. On advice from medical direction, you may administer small doses of morphine sulfate to reduce patient anxiety. After confirming the absence of GI bleeding, medical direction may also prescribe anticoagulants to prevent clot formation and/or to speed clot dissolution. If the administration of a vasopressor is indicated by low blood pressure, then dopamine may be prescribed. In such cases, remember to titrate the dopamine to a desirable blood pressure.

The risk of death from pulmonary embolism is greatest in the first few hours. As a result, rapid transport is essential. Position the patient in an upright position and avoid lifting the patient by the legs or knees, which may dislodge thrombi in the lower extremities. During transport, continue to monitor changes in skin color, pulse oximetry, and changes in breathing rate and rhythm. Your field assessment and interventions can save the patient's life and guide the hospital physician in a direction that will result in an accurate diagnosis and rapid treatment.

Pulmonary Edema. Pulmonary edema causes severe dyspnea associated with congestion. Other signs and symptoms include rapid labored breathing, cough with blood-stained sputum, cyanosis, and cold extremities. Physical examination usually reveals the presence of moist crackles and accessory muscle use. Severe cases will exhibit rhonchi.

©2013 Pearson Education, Inc.
Paramedic Care: Principles & Practice, Vol. 6, 4th Ed.

Treatment is directed toward altering the cause of the condition. The existence of pulmonary edema can be life threatening and is often the symptom of a fatal cardiovascular disease.

Lung Cancer. Treatment of lung cancer occurs in a hospital setting. However, you may be called to assist with the follow-up home care or, in terminal stages, in a hospice situation.

Cardiovascular Disorders pp. 160–162

In conducting your history, determine the patient's level of cardiovascular fitness, changes in exercise tolerance, recent diet history, use of medications, and use of cigarettes and/or alcohol. Ask questions about breathing difficulty, especially at night, and evidence of palpitations, flutter, or skipped beats.

In performing the physical exam, look for hypertension and orthostatic hypotension (a decrease in blood pressure and an increase in heart rate when rising from a seated or supine position). Watch for dehydration or dependent edema. When taking an elderly patient's blood pressure, consider checking both arms. Routinely determine pulses in all the extremities. In auscultating the patient, remember that a bruit or noise in the neck, abdomen, or groin indicates a high probability of carotid, aortorenal, or peripheral vascular disease. Keep in mind, too, that heart sounds are generally softer in the elderly, probably because of a thickening of lung tissue between the heart and chest wall.

In evaluating the problem, recall the cardiovascular disorders commonly found in elderly patients. They include angina pectoris, myocardial infarction, heart failure, arrhythmias, aortic dissection, aneurysm, hypertension, and syncope.

Angina Pectoris. Angina pectoris literally means "pain in the chest." However, the pain of angina is actually felt in only about 10 percent to 20 percent of elderly patients. The changes in sensory nerves, combined with the myocardial changes of aging, make dyspnea a more likely symptom of angina than pain.

Angina develops when narrowing of coronary vessels as a result of plaque or vasospasm leads to an inability to meet the oxygen demands of the heart muscle. The heart muscle usually responds by sending out pain signals, which represent a buildup of lactic acid. In an elderly patient, exercise intolerance is a key symptom of angina. In obtaining a history, you should ask the patient about sudden changes in routine. In addition, inquire about any increased stresses on the heart, such as anemia, infection, arrhythmias, and thyroid changes.

General prevention strategies in the elderly are similar to those in young patients. Blood pressure control combined with diet, exercise, and smoking modifications reduces the risk in all groups.

Myocardial Infarction. A myocardial infarction is most commonly triggered by some form of physical exertion or a preexisting heart disease. Because of the high mortality associated with myocardial infarctions in the elderly, early detection and emergency management are critical.

Heart Failure. Signs and symptoms of heart failure vary. In most patients, regardless of age, some form of edema exists. However, edema in the elderly can indicate a range of problems, including musculoskeletal injury. Assessment findings specific to the elderly include: fatigue (left failure), two-pillow orthopnea, dyspnea on exertion, dry and hacking cough progressing to productive cough, dependent edema (right failure), nocturia, anorexia, hepatomegaly, and ascites.

Nonpharmacologic management of heart failure includes modifications in diet (e.g., less fat and cholesterol), exercise, and reduction in weight, if necessary. Pharmacologic management may include treatment with diuretics, vasodilators, antihypertensive agents, or inotropic agents. Check to see whether the patient is already on any of these medications and if the patient is compliant with scheduled doses.

Arrhythmias. Treatment considerations depend on the type of arrhythmia. Patients may already have a pacemaker in place. In such cases, keep in mind that pacemakers have a low but significant rate of complications such as a failed battery, fibrosis around the catheter site, lead fracture, or electrode dislodgment. In a number of situations, drug therapy may be indicated. Whenever you discover an arrhythmia, remember that an abnormal or disordered heart rhythm may be the only clinical finding in an elderly patient suffering acute myocardial infarction.

Aortic Dissection/Aneurysms. The aneurysm may appear as a pulsatile mass in a patient with a normal girth, but lack of an identifiable mass does not eliminate this condition. Patients may present with tearing abdominal pain or unexplained low back pain. Pulses in the legs are diminished or absent and the lower extremities feel cold to the touch. The patient may experience sensory abnormalities such as numbness, tingling, or pain in the legs. The patient may fall when attempting to stand.

Treatment of an aneurysm depends on its size, location, and the severity of the condition. In the case of thoracic aortic dissection, continuous IV infusion and/or administration of drug therapy to lower the arterial pressure and to diminish the velocity of left ventricle contraction may be indicated. Rapid transport is essential, especially for the older patient who most commonly requires care and observation in an intensive care unit.

Hypertension. Hypertension is often a silent disease that produces no clinically obvious signs or symptoms. It may be associated with nonspecific complaints such as headache, tinnitus, epistaxis, slow tremors, or nausea and vomiting. An acute onset of high blood pressure without any kidney involvement is often a telltale indicator of thyroid disease.

Management of hypertension depends on its severity and the existence of other conditions. For example, hypertension is often treated with beta-blockers—medications that are contraindicated in patients with chronic obstructive lung disease, asthma, or heart block greater than first degree. Diuretics, another common drug used in treating hypertension, should be prescribed with care for patients on digitalis. Keep in mind that centrally acting agents are more likely to produce negative side effects in the elderly. Unlike younger patients, the elderly may experience depression, forgetfulness, sleep problems, or vivid dreams and/or hallucinations.

Syncope. Each elderly patient presents a unique challenge in terms of assessment and management. You will need to tailor your management plan to fit a patient's illness, injury, and overall general health.

Neurologic Disorders   pp. 162–165
In the field, it is often impossible to distinguish the cause of an altered mental status. Even so, you should carry out a thorough assessment. Administer supplemental oxygen if the patient is hypoxic. As soon as practical, obtain a blood glucose level to exclude hypoglycemia as a possible cause. Overall, the approach to the elderly patient with altered mental status is the same as that for any other patient presenting with similar symptoms.

Cerebrovascular Disease (Stroke/TIAs). Because of the various kinds of strokes, signs and symptoms can present in many ways: altered mental status, coma, paralysis, slurred speech, a change in mood, and seizures. Stroke should be highly suspect in any elderly patient with a sudden change in mental status.

Whenever you suspect a stroke, it is essential that you complete the Los Angeles Prehospital Stroke Screen or Cincinnati Prehospital Stroke Scale for later comparison in the emergency department. Fibrinolytic agents administered to a patient suffering an occlusive (ischemic) stroke can decrease the severity of damage if administered within 4.5 hours of onset. Rapid transport is essential for avoiding brain damage or limiting its extent. In the case of stroke, "time is brain tissue."

Seizures. Often the cause of the seizure cannot be determined in the field. As a result, treat the condition as a life-threatening emergency and transport as quickly as possible to eliminate the possibility of stroke. If the patient has fallen during a seizure, check for evidence of trauma and treat accordingly.

Dizziness/Vertigo. Vertigo results from so many factors that it is often hard, even for the physician, to determine the actual cause. Any factor that impairs visual input, inner-ear function, peripheral sensory input, or the central nervous system can cause dizziness. In addition, alcohol and many prescription drugs can cause dizziness. So can hypoglycemia in its early stages. It is virtually impossible to distinguish dizziness, syncope, and presyncope in the prehospital setting.

Delirium. The presentation of delirium varies greatly and can change rapidly during assessment. Common signs and symptoms include the acute onset of anxiety, an inability to focus, disordered thinking, irritability, inappropriate behavior, fearfulness, excessive energy, or psychotic behavior such as hallucinations or paranoia. Aphasia or speaking errors and/or prominent slurring of speech may be present. Normal patterns of eating and sleeping are almost always disrupted.

In distinguishing between delirium and dementia, err on the side of delirium. The condition is often caused by life-threatening, but reversible, conditions. Causes of delirium, such as infections, drug toxicity, and electrolyte imbalances, generally have a good prognosis if identified quickly and managed promptly.

©2013 Pearson Education, Inc.
Paramedic Care: Principles & Practice, Vol. 6, 4th Ed.

Dementia. Signs and symptoms of dementia include progressive disorientation, shortened attention span, aphasia or nonsense talking, and hallucinations. Dementia often hampers treatment through the patient's inability to communicate, and it can exhaust caregivers. In moderate to severe cases, you will need to rely on the caregiver for information. Remain alert to signs of abuse or neglect, which occurs in a disproportionate number of elderly suffering from dementia.

Alzheimer's Disease. Alzheimer's disease generally occurs in stages, each with different signs and symptoms. These stages include:

- Early stage. Characterized by loss of recent memory, inability to learn new material, mood swings, and personality changes. Patients may believe someone is plotting against them when they lose items or forget things. Aggression or hostility is common. Poor judgment is evident.
- Intermediate stage. Characterized by a complete inability to learn new material; wandering, particularly at night; increased falls; and loss of ability for self-care, including bathing and use of the toilet.
- Terminal stage. Characterized by an inability to walk and regression to infant stage, including the loss of bowel and bladder function. Eventually the patient loses the ability to eat and swallow.

Families caring for an Alzheimer's patient at home also present signs of stress. Remember to treat both the Alzheimer's patient and the family and/or caregivers with respect and compassion. Evaluate the needs of the family and make an appropriate report at your facility. Support groups are available to assist families.

Parkinson's Disease. It is impossible in a field setting to distinguish primary and secondary Parkinson's disease. The most common initial sign of a Parkinson's disorder is a resting tremor combined with a pill-rolling motion. As the disease progresses, muscles become more rigid and movements become slower and/or more jerky. In some cases, patients may find their movements halted while carrying out some routine task. Their feet may feel "frozen to the ground." Gaits becomes shuffled with short steps and unexpected bursts of speed, often to avoid falling. Kyphotic deformity is a hallmark of the disease.

Patients with Parkinson's disease commonly develop mask-like faces devoid of all expression. They speak in slow, monotone voices. Difficulties in communication, coupled with a loss of mobility, often lead to anxiety and depression.

There is no known cure for Parkinson's disease, with the exception of drug-induced secondary Parkinson's disorders. Exercise may help maintain physical activity or teach the patient adaptive strategies. In calls involving a Parkinson's patient, observe for the conditions that involved the EMS system, such as a fall or the inability to move. Manage treatable conditions and transport as needed.

Metabolic and Endocrine Disorders   pp. 165–166

Diabetes Mellitus. Management of diabetic and hypoglycemic emergencies for the elderly is generally the same as for any other patient. Do not rule out alcohol as a complicating factor, especially in cases of hypoglycemia. In addition, remember that diabetes places the elderly at increased risk of other complications, including atherosclerosis, delayed healing, retinopathy, blindness, altered renal function, and severe peripheral vascular disease, leading to foot ulcers and even amputations.

Thyroid Disorders. Less than 33 percent of the elderly present with typical signs and symptoms of hypothyroidism. When they do, their complaints are often attributed to aging. Common nonspecific complaints in the elderly include mental confusion, anorexia, falls, incontinence, and decreased mobility. Some patients also experience an increase in muscle or joint pain. Treatment involves thyroid hormone replacement.

Hyperthyroidism is less common among the elderly but may result from medication errors such as an overdose of thyroid hormone replacement. The typical symptom of heat intolerance is often present. Otherwise, hyperthyroidism presents atypically in the elderly. Common nonspecific features or complaints include atrial fibrillation, failure to thrive (weight loss and apathy combined), abdominal distress, diarrhea, exhaustion, and depression.

The diagnosis and treatment of thyroid disorders does not take place in the field. Elderly patients with known thyroid problems should be encouraged to go to the hospital for medical evaluation.

Gastrointestinal Disorders   pp. 166–167

Regardless of the complaint, remember that prompt management of a GI emergency is essential for young and old alike. For the elderly, there is a significant risk of hemorrhage and shock. There is a tendency to take GI patients less seriously than those suffering moderate or severe external hemorrhage. This is a serious mistake. Patients with gastrointestinal complaints, especially the elderly, should be managed aggressively. Keep in mind that older patients are far more intolerant of hypotension and anoxia than younger patients are. Treatment should include airway management, support of breathing and circulation, supplemental oxygen therapy if the patient is hypoxic, IV fluid replacement with a crystalloid solution, and rapid transport.

GI Hemorrhage. Signs of significant gastrointestinal blood loss include the presence of "coffee-grounds" emesis; black, tar-like stools (melena); obvious blood in the emesis or stool; orthostatic hypotension; pulse greater than 100 (unless the patient is on beta-blockers); and confusion. Gastrointestinal bleeding in the elderly may result in such complications as a recent increase in angina symptoms, congestive heart failure, weakness, or dyspnea.

Bowel Obstruction. The patient will typically complain of diffuse abdominal pain, bloating, nausea, and vomiting. The abdomen may feel distended when palpated. Bowel sounds may be hypoactive or absent. If the obstruction has been present for a prolonged period of time, the patient may have fever, weakness, shock, and various electrolyte disturbances.

Mesenteric Ischemia/Infarct. The primary symptom of a bowel infarct is pain out of proportion to the physical exam. Signs include bloody diarrhea, some tachycardia, and abdominal distention.

The patient is at great risk for shock because the dead bowel attracts interstitial and intravascular fluids, thus removing them from use. Necrotic products are released to the peritoneal cavity, leading to a massive infection. The prognosis is poor due, in part, to the decreased physiological reserves of the older patient.

Skin Disorders   pp. 167–168

Skin Diseases. In treating skin disorders, remember that many conditions may be drug induced.

Beta-blockers, for example, can worsen psoriasis, which occurs in about 3 percent of elderly patients. Question patients about their medications, keeping in mind that certain prescription drugs (e.g., penicillins and sulfonamides) and some OTC drugs can cause skin eruptions. Also ask about topical home remedies, such as alcohol or soaps, that may cause or worsen the disorder. Find out whether the patient is compliant with prescribed topical treatments. Finally, remember that some drugs and topical medications commonly used to treat skin disorders in the young can worsen or cause other problems for the elderly. Antihistamines and corticosteroids are two to three times more likely to provoke adverse reactions in the elderly than in younger adults.

Pressure Ulcers (Decubitus Ulcers). To reduce the development of pressure ulcers or to alleviate their condition, you can take these steps:

- Assist the patient in changing position frequently, especially during extended transport, to reduce the length of time pressure is placed on any one point.
- Use a pull sheet to move the patient, reducing the likelihood of friction.
- Reduce the possibility of shearing by padding areas of skin prior to movement.
- Unless a life-threatening condition is present, take time to clean and dry areas of excessive moisture, such as urinary or fecal incontinence and excessive perspiration.
- Clean ulcers with normal saline solution and cover with hydrocolloid or hydrogel dressings, if available. With severe ulcers, pack with loosely woven gauze moistened with normal saline.

Musculoskeletal Disorders   pp. 168–170

Osteoarthritis. Osteoarthritis in the elderly presents initially as joint pain, worsened by exercise and improved by rest. As the disease progresses, pain may be accompanied by diminished mobility, joint deformity, and crepitus or grating sensations. Late signs include tenderness on palpation or during passive motion.

The most effective treatment involves management before the disability develops or worsens. Prevention strategies include stretching exercises and activities that strengthen stress-absorbing ligaments. Immobilization, even for short periods, can accelerate the condition. Drug therapy is usually aimed at

©2013 Pearson Education, Inc.
Paramedic Care: Principles & Practice, Vol. 6, 4th Ed.

lessening pain and/or inflammation. Surgery is usually the last resort after more conservative methods have failed.

Osteoporosis. Unless a bone density test is conducted, persons with osteoporosis are usually asymptomatic until a fracture occurs. The precipitating event can be as slight as turning over in bed, carrying a package, or even a forceful sneeze.

Management includes prevention of fractures through exercise and drug therapy, such as the administration of calcium, vitamin D, estrogen, and other medications or minerals. Once the condition occurs, pain management also becomes a consideration.

Ankylosing Spondylitis. EMS providers called to care for a victim of AS must remember that their patient's spine is inflexible and cannot be moved. Furthermore, the fused spine can be extremely fragile and subject to fracture, with resultant spinal cord injury. Numerous EMS techniques must be modified to accommodate patients with AS. These include airway management techniques, splinting techniques, and transport considerations. Because most AS patients have spinal flexion, it is important to adequately pad underneath the patient's head, neck, and upper back with pillow or pillows. Likewise, airway management techniques must be applied without extending the neck. Airway devices that do not require visualization should be considered instead of endotracheal intubation, with cricothyrotomy used as a last resort.

Renal Disorders p. 170

Urinary Disorders. Signs or symptoms of a UTI range from cloudy, foul-smelling urine to the typical complaints of bladder pain and frequent urination. Urosepsis presents as an acute process, including fever, chills, abdominal discomfort, and other signs of septic shock. The septicemia generally begins within 24 to 72 hours after catheterization or cystoscopy.

Treatment of urosepsis commonly includes placement of a large-bore IV catheter for administration of fluids and parenteral antibiotics. Diagnosis of urosepsis is based on history and other physical findings. Prompt transport is critical. The prognosis for elderly patients with urosepsis is poor, with a mortality rate of approximately 30 percent. Maintenance of fluid balance, as well as adequate blood pressure, is essential.

15. **Adapt equipment and techniques of management to meet the needs of geriatric patients.** p. 152

People become less like one another as they age. Therefore, each elderly patient presents a unique challenge in terms of assessment and management. You will need to tailor your management plan to fit a patient's illness, injury, and overall general health. Because of the potential for rapid deterioration among the elderly, you must quickly spot conditions requiring rapid transport.

As with any other patient, your first concern is the primary assessment. Remain alert at all times for changes in an elderly patient's neurologic status, vital signs, and general cardiac status. (Management of specific disorders and the administration of medications to the elderly are covered in other sections of this chapter.)

In general, remember that transport to a hospital is often more stressful for the elderly than to any other age group, except for the very young. Avoid lights and sirens in all but the most serious cases, such as when you suspect a pulmonary embolism or bowel infarction. A calm, smooth transport helps to reduce patient anxiety—and the resulting strain that anxiety places on an elderly patient's heart.

Provide emotional support at every phase of the call. Nearly any serious illness or injury in the elderly can provoke a sense of impending doom. Death is a very real possibility to this age group. To help reduce patient fears, keep these guidelines in mind:

- Encourage patients to express their feelings.
- Do not trivialize their fears.
- Acknowledge nonverbal messages.
- Avoid questions that are judgmental.
- Confirm what the patient says.

- Recall all you have learned about communicating with the elderly, thus avoiding communication breakdowns.
- Assure patients that you understand that they are adults on an equal footing with their care providers, including you.

16. Recognize indications of abuse or neglect of a geriatric patient. p. 177

Abuse of the elderly is as big of a problem in our society as child abuse and neglect. Geriatric abuse is defined as a syndrome in which an elderly person has received serious physical or psychological injury from family members or other caregivers.

The profile for the potential geriatric abuser may often show a great deal of life stress. In many cases, sleep deprivation, marital discord, financial problems, and work-related problems exist.

Signs and symptoms of geriatric abuse and neglect are often obvious. Unexplained trauma is usually the primary presentation. The average abused patient is older than 80 and has multiple medical problems, such as cancer, congestive heart failure, heart disease, and incontinence. Senile dementia is often present.

17. Communicate relevant patient information orally and in writing when transferring care of the geriatric patient to hospital personnel. pp. 140–179

During your classroom, clinical, and field training, you will interact and communicate with real and simulated patients, family members, bystanders, other responders, and hospital personnel. When performing a general health assessment, take into account the patient's living situation, level of activity, network of social support, level of independence, medication history (both prescription and nonprescription), and sleep patterns. In addition to the information presented in this chapter, you will use the information from Volume 1, Chapter 9: EMS System Communications; Volume 1, Chapter 10: Documentation; and Volume 3, Chapter 3: Therapeutic Communications to effectively communicate and document assessment findings, patient management, and patient response to care. Continue to refine these skills once your training ends and you begin your career as a paramedic.

Case Study Review

Reread the case study on pages 138 to 139 in Paramedic Care: Special Patients; *then, read the following discussion.*

This case study draws attention to the importance of recognizing the vital lives led by elderly people and the need to take their complaints seriously, rather than dismissing them as normal age-related changes.

The case study puts you in the position of a paramedic who decides to mentor a student intern about the treatment of elderly patients. At the end of the call, the intern is asked: "So, Andy, do you want to talk about what went right with this call and what we could have done better while we restock the ambulance?"

So let's discuss it! The complaint of abdominal pain can be caused by many different factors, most of which cannot not be resolved in a prehospital setting. Even so, after reading the text, you now know that the most frequent gastrointestinal emergency in the elderly is GI bleeding, a condition that can place the elderly at a significant risk of hypovolemia and shock. The elderly are also far more intolerant of hypotension and anoxia than younger patients. Any GI emergency should be aggressively managed.

In this case, the initial assessment ruled out an immediate life threat. The general impression was that of an elderly woman with severe abdominal pain. As noted, the pain was out of proportion to the physical exam—a symptom suggestive of mesenteric infarct. Care steps included administration of high-concentration oxygen, IV fluid replacement therapy with a crystalloid solution, and, most important, rapid transport.

It was correct to place the patient on a cardiac monitor. An ECG of atrial fibrillation is common in elderly patients. Based on the patient's vital signs, Mrs. Hildegaard seemed to be tolerating the dysrhythmias. The monitor helped show that the pain was not cardiac related, though complications could result, depending on preexisting medical conditions.

It might have been helpful to inquire in more detail about any other GI distress experienced by the patient, such as diarrhea, vomiting, and nausea. Also, a pulse oximeter might have been useful to measure the patient's oxygen saturation en route to the hospital. However, considering the patient's presentation, she was managed appropriately.

Andy's quip about too many beers and a taco provided a "teachable moment" in that it corrected a mistaken attitude about the aging process—the idea that an elderly patient might not live like a younger counterpart. In fact, it would have been relevant to ask just what the patient ate—and drank—at dinner. It also highlighted the problem of alcohol abuse among the elderly. They are not only exposed to the stresses of aging, but age-related systemic changes and medical problems make it more difficult for them to metabolize alcohol and many other drugs. Thus it would have also been relevant to ask whether Mrs. Hildegaard consumed alcohol on a regular basis.

Content Self-Evaluation

MULTIPLE CHOICE

_____ 1. All of the following are responsible for the growing number of elderly people in the United States—and the projected increase in the number of elderly patients treated by EMS services—EXCEPT
    A. an increase in the mean survival rate of older persons.
    B. an increase in the birth rate.
    C. the absence of major wars.
    D. improved health care.
    E. improved standard of living.

_____ 2. The scientific study of the effects of aging and of age-related diseases on humans is known as
    A. geriatrics.   **D.** eldercare.
    B. ageism.   **E.** gerontotherapeutics.
    C. gerontology.

_____ 3. The elderly often do not reveal problems behind the chief complaints because they
    A. fear the loss of their independence.
    B. consider the problems "normal" for their age.
    C. don't want to burden others with their problems.
    D. do not want to be treated as helpless human beings.
    E. all of the above.

_____ 4. A living arrangement in which the elderly live in, but do not own, individual apartments or rooms and receive selective services is known as
    A. a nursing home.   **D.** a personal-care home.
    B. a life-care community.   **E.** a hospice.
    C. congregate care.

_____ 5. Drawbacks to living in an adult community or nursing home setting include all of the following, EXCEPT
    A. loss of independence.
    B. exposure to illnesses found in the institutional setting.
    C. a lack of contact with young people.
    D. increased risk of criminal activities.
    E. low-quality or inadequate staff.

_____ 6. A deterioration in independence is a function of aging and should be treated as such by the paramedic.
    A. True
    B. False

7. When confronted with multiple decision makers during the care of an elderly patient, you should usually honor the wishes of the
   A. caregiver.
   B. family members.
   C. personal-care aide.
   D. patient.
   E. spouse or partner.

8. The largest share of public funding for long-term care of the elderly is provided by
   A. the Veterans Administration.
   B. Medicaid.
   C. Medicare.
   D. private insurance.
   E. health maintenance organizations.

9. Health care endeavors supported by many senior centers include
   A. blood pressure monitoring.
   B. transport to clinics.
   C. Meals on Wheels.
   D. flu shots.
   E. all of the above.

10. All of the following provide significant advocacy for the elderly, EXCEPT
    A. AA.
    B. AARP.
    C. Alzheimer's Association.
    D. Association for Senior Citizens.
    E. Department of Health.

11. The usage of multiple medications in the elderly patient is known as
    A. polyprognosis.
    B. mulipharmaceuticals.
    C. polypharmacy.
    D. polyphasia.
    E. multimedicinal.

12. Common complaints and injuries to the elderly include
    A. falls, weakness, and syncope.
    B. fractures, drowning, and diabetes.
    C. stab wounds, croup, and nausea.
    D. motor vehicle collisions, meningitis, and poisoning.
    E. fever, epiglottitis, and febrile seizures.

13. When compared with younger patients, the elderly experience fewer adverse drug reactions.
    A. True
    B. False

14. Drugs concentrate more readily in the plasma and tissues of elderly patients because of
    A. diminished neurologic function.
    B. increased body fluid.
    C. atrophy of organs.
    D. more efficient compensatory mechanisms.
    E. increased renal function.

15. Factors that can decrease medication compliance in the elderly include all of the following, EXCEPT
    A. limited mobility.
    B. fear of toxicity.
    C. child-proof containers.
    D. multiple-compartment pill boxes.
    E. sensory impairment.

16. Factors that can increase medication compliance in the elderly include
    A. compliance counseling.
    B. a belief that an illness is serious.
    C. clear, simple directions.
    D. blister-pack packaging.
    E. all of the above.

17. A lack of mobility can have detrimental physical and emotional effects on the elderly.
    A. True
    B. False

©2013 Pearson Education, Inc.
Paramedic Care: Principles & Practice, Vol. 6, 4th Ed.

18. Which of the following is the leading cause of accidental deaths among the elderly?
A. Drownings
B. Fall-related injuries
C. Motor vehicle collisions
D. Gunshot wounds
E. Poisonings

19. Intrinsic factors that can cause an elderly person to fall include all of the following, EXCEPT
A. dizziness.
B. slippery floors.
C. decreased mental status.
D. impaired vision.
E. CNS problems.

20. Extrinsic factors that can cause an elderly person to fall include
A. an altered gait.
B. a sense of weakness.
C. a lack of hand rails.
D. use of certain medications.
E. a history of repeated falls.

21. The inability to retain urine or feces because of loss of sphincter control or because of cerebral or spinal lesions is called
A. diarrhea.
B. involuntary elimination.
C. diuresis.
D. incontinence.
E. uremia.

22. In elderly people with cerebrovascular disease or impaired baroreceptor reflexes, efforts to force a bowel movement can lead to a transient ischemic attack.
A. True
B. False

23. Which of the following drugs can cause constipation?
A. Diuretics
B. Opioids
C. Anticholinergics
D. Cation-containing agents
E. All of the above

24. All of the following factors play a part in forming a general assessment of the elderly patient EXCEPT
A. average cost of rent.
B. medication history.
C. living situations.
D. sleep patterns.
E. level of activity.

25. One of the most common reasons that elderly patients underestimate the severity of a primary medical problem is that they have a(n)
A. shrinkage of structures in the ear.
B. clouding and thickening of lenses in the eyes.
C. lowered sensitivity to pain.
D. deterioration of the teeth and gums.
E. altered sense of taste.

26. Conditions that may complicate or discourage eating among the elderly include
A. breathing or respiratory problems.
B. psychological disorders.
C. poor dental care.
D. alcohol or drug abuse
E. all of the above.

27. An eating disorder marked by excessive fasting found in the elderly and other age groups is called
A. diverticulitis.
B. dysphagia.
C. anorexia nervosa.
D. bulimia.
E. dehydration.

28. Which of the following is a by-product of malnutrition?
A. Electrolyte abnormalities
B. Dehydration
C. Vitamin deficiencies
D. Hyperglycemia
E. All of the above

_____ **29.** The elderly are more prone to environmental thermal problems due to changes in the sweat glands.
A. True
B. False

_____ **30.** A medical condition in which eye pressure increases and ultimately diminishes sight is known as
A. Meniere's disease.
B. tinnitus.
C. cataracts.
D. glaucoma.
E. retinitis.

_____ **31.** A disease of the inner ear characterized by vertigo, nerve deafness, and a roar or buzzing in the ear is called
A. Meniere's disease.
B. tinnitus.
C. cataracts.
D. glaucoma.
E. cerumen.

_____ **32.** To improve communication with an elderly patient, you should try to
A. display verbal and nonverbal signs of concern.
B. dim the room lights.
C. avoid looking directly into the patient's eyes.
D. first talk to family members, then the patient.
E. remain as quiet as possible.

_____ **33.** Both senility and organic brain syndrome may manifest themselves as
A. distractibility.
B. excitability.
C. hostility.
D. restlessness.
E. all of the above.

_____ **34.** When assessing an elderly person, if he is confused or disoriented, you can conclude that the patient is senile.
A. True
B. False

_____ **35.** Dependent edema may be caused by inactivity, not just congestive heart failure.
A. True
B. False

_____ **36.** To help reduce an elderly patient's fears, you should
A. downplay the patient's fears.
B. ignore nonverbal messages.
C. discourage the expression of feelings.
D. confirm what the patient has said.
E. instruct the patient to calm down.

_____ **37.** Age-related changes to the respiratory system include all of the following, EXCEPT
A. increased chest wall compliance.
B. diminished breathing capacity.
C. reduced strength and endurance.
D. increased air trapping.
E. loss of lung elasticity.

_____ **38.** The inactivity of the _____ make the elderly more prone to respiratory infection.
A. gag reflex
B. alveoli
C. cilia
D. bronchioles
E. vagal response

_____ **39.** In treating respiratory disorders in the elderly patient, do not fluid overload.
A. True
B. False

©2013 Pearson Education, Inc.
Paramedic Care: Principles & Practice, Vol. 6, 4th Ed.

40. An increase in the size and bulk of the left ventricle wall in some elderly patients is an example of
- **A.** kyphosis.
- **B.** anoxia hypoxemia.
- **C.** hypertrophy.
- **D.** fibrosis.
- **E.** Marfan's syndrome.

41. In managing elderly patients with complaints related to the cardiovascular system, take all of the following steps, EXCEPT
- **A.** monitor the ECG.
- **B.** administer oxygen if the patient is hypoxic.
- **C.** walk the patient slowly to the rig.
- **D.** remain empathetic to the patient's fears.
- **E.** start an IV for possible medication administration.

42. All of the following are age-related changes to the nervous system, EXCEPT
- **A.** decreased reaction time.
- **B.** increased brain weight.
- **C.** impaired balance.
- **D.** shrinkage of brain tissue.
- **E.** recent memory loss.

43. The elderly are less susceptible to subdural hematomas than younger people.
- **A.** True
- **B.** False

44. Age-related changes in the gastrointestinal system include all of the following, EXCEPT
- **A.** impaired swallowing.
- **B.** diminished digestive functions.
- **C.** decreased liver efficiency.
- **D.** a predisposition to choking.
- **E.** increased gastric secretions.

45. A protrusion of the stomach upward into the mediastinal cavity through the diaphragm is known as
- **A.** a hiatal hernia.
- **B.** Marfan's syndrome.
- **C.** a diaphragmatic hernia.
- **D.** an inguinal hernia.
- **E.** an epigastric hernia.

46. In the elderly, injury to the skin is often more severe than in younger patients and healing time is increased. As a rule, the elderly are at a higher risk of
- **A** secondary infection.
- **B.** skin tumors.
- **C.** drug-inducted eruptions.
- **D.** fungal or viral infections.
- **E.** all of the above.

47. The elderly have a greater risk of trauma-related complications due to a decrease in blood volume.
- **A.** True
- **B.** False

48. An exaggeration of the normal posterior curvature of the spine is called
- **A.** scoliosis.
- **B.** kyphosis.
- **C.** fibrosis.
- **D.** hypertrophy.
- **E.** spondylosis.

49. Reasons that the elderly develop pneumonia more frequently than younger people include all of the following, EXCEPT a(n)
- **A.** decreased immune response.
- **B.** increased pulmonary function.
- **C.** abnormal or ineffective cough reflex.
- **D.** decreased activity of mucociliary cells.
- **E.** increased colonization of the pharynx by gram-negative bacteria.

50. An elderly patient in an institutional setting is up to 50 times more likely to contract pneumonia than an elderly patient receiving home care.
    A. True
    B. False

51. The usual signs and symptoms of COPD include
    A. cough and wheezing.
    B. dyspnea and tachypnea.
    C. exercise intolerance.
    D. pleuritic chest pain.
    E. all of the above.

52. The most effective prevention of COPD involves
    A. elimination of smoking.
    B. lowering blood sugar.
    C. reducing physical activity.
    D. lowering blood pressure.
    E. use of supplemental oxygen.

53. Your elderly patient is complaining of acute onset of sharp chest pain and shortness of breath. The patient was recently released from the hospital for a leg fracture. What is the most likely suspected disorder?
    A. pneumonia
    B. pulmonary embolism
    C. heart attack
    D. COPD
    E. pulmonary edema

54. Although all of the following can contribute to a pulmonary embolism, the condition is most frequently caused by
    A. fat.
    B. bone marrow.
    C. blood clots.
    D. tumor cells.
    E. air.

55. The leading cause of death in the elderly is
    A. pneumonia.
    B. stroke.
    C. cardiovascular disease.
    D. Alzheimer's disease.
    E. COPD.

56. The heart sounds in an elderly patient are generally louder than those in a young patient.
    A. True
    B. False

57. All of the following are atypical presentations of a myocardial infarction that may be seen in the elderly, EXCEPT
    A. syncope.
    B. tearing chest pain.
    C. dyspnea.
    D. neck or dental pain.
    E. exercise intolerance.

58. Assessment findings specific to the elderly such as anorexia, nocturia, dependent edema, and hepatomegaly may be found in a patient with
    A. a pulmonary embolism.
    B. heart failure.
    C. hypertension.
    D. an aneurysm.
    E. syncope.

59. An abnormal dilation of a blood vessel, usually an artery, due to a congenital defect or weakness in the wall of the vessel is called
    A. an aneurysm.
    B. an infarct.
    C. thrombosis.
    D. an embolism.
    E. a hernia.

60. A series of symptoms resulting from decreased blood flow to the brain that is caused by a sudden decrease in cardiac output from a heart block is known as
    A. autonomic dysfunction.
    B. Stokes-Adams syndrome.
    C. sick sinus syndrome.
    D. dying heart muscle.
    E. Marfan's syndrome.

_____ **61.** Injury to or death of brain tissue resulting from interruption of cerebral blood flow and oxygenation is called a(n):
- **A.** subarachnoid hemorrhage.
- **B.** autonomic dysfunction.
- **C.** TIA.
- **D.** stroke.
- **E.** intracerebral hemorrhage.

_____ **62.** Common causes of seizures in the elderly include all of the following, EXCEPT
- **A.** head trauma.
- **B.** alcohol withdrawal.
- **C.** spinal injury.
- **D.** stroke.
- **E.** hypoglycemia.

_____ **63.** A chronic, degenerative disease that attacks the brain and results in impaired memory, thinking, and behavior is called
- **A.** dementia.
- **B.** Parkinson's disease.
- **C.** delirium.
- **D.** Alzheimer's disease.
- **E.** aphasia.

_____ **64.** A chronic, degenerative nervous disease characterized by tremors, muscular weakness and rigidity, and loss of postural reflexes is called
- **A.** Parkinson's disease.
- **B.** Shy-Drager syndrome.
- **C.** Alzheimer's disease.
- **D.** sick sinus syndrome.
- **E.** a generalized tonic-clonic seizure.

_____ **65.** All of the following are forms of upper GI bleeding, EXCEPT
- **A.** a Mallory-Weiss tear.
- **B.** ischemic colitis.
- **C.** esophageal varices.
- **D.** gastritis.
- **E.** peptic ulcer disease.

_____ **66.** An example of a lower GI bleeding is
- **A.** a Mallory-Weiss tear.
- **B.** diverticulosis.
- **C.** peptic ulcer disease.
- **D.** a bowel obstruction.
- **E.** a mesenteric infarct.

_____ **67.** An abnormal dilation of veins in the lower esophagus common in patients with cirrhosis of the liver is called esophageal varices.
- **A.** True
- **B.** False

_____ **68.** An inflammation of the colon resulting from impaired or decreased blood supply is called
- **A.** diverticulosis.
- **B.** ischemic colitis.
- **C.** arterio-venous malformation.
- **D.** colostomy.
- **E.** gastritis.

_____ **69.** The acute skin eruption caused by a reactivation of the latent varicella virus that peaks between ages 50 and 70 is known as
- **A.** shingles.
- **B.** pruritus.
- **C.** maceration.
- **D.** herpes zoster.
- **E.** both A and D.

_____ **70.** When transporting an elderly patient with pressure ulcers, you should encourage the patient to remain still.
- **A.** True
- **B.** False

_____ **71.** Risk factors for osteoporosis include all of the following, EXCEPT
- **A.** African or Latino ancestry.
- **B.** low body weight.
- **C.** late menopause.
- **D.** family history of fractures.
- **E.** use of caffeine, alcohol, and cigarettes.

_____ 72. In general, the kidney loses approximately one-third of its weight between the ages of 30 and 80.
   A. True
   B. False

_____ 73. All of the following are signs and symptoms of hypothermia in an elderly patient, EXCEPT
   A. confusion.
   B. slow speech.
   C. shivering.
   D. skin cool to the touch.
   E. sleepiness.

_____ 74. Lidocaine is the most widely used cardiac glycoside for the management of congestive heart failure, atrial fibrillation, atrial flutter, paroxysmal atrial tachycardia, and cardiogenic shock.
   A. True
   B. False

_____ 75. Arrhythmias commonly associated with digoxin toxicity include all of the following, EXCEPT
   A. atrial fibrillation.
   B. third-degree heart block.
   C. sinoatrial exit block.
   D. ventricular fibrillation.
   E. sinoatrial arrest.

_____ 76. The most common adverse drug effect that occurs in the elderly is
   A. lidocaine underdose.
   B. digoxin toxicity.
   C. furosemide overdose.
   D. lithium toxicity.
   E. morphine addiction.

_____ 77. Factors that contribute to substance abuse among the elderly include
   A. multiple prescriptions.
   B. malnutrition.
   C. loneliness.
   D. age-related changes.
   E. all of the above.

_____ 78. The elderly who become physically and/or psychologically dependent upon drugs (or alcohol) are more likely to seek help than those in other age groups.
   A. True
   B. False

_____ 79. The leading cause of suicide among the elderly is
   A. chronic illness.
   B. unrelieved pain.
   C. living in a youth-oriented society.
   D. financial problems.
   E. depression.

_____ 80. One of the best indicators of shock in an elderly patient is
   A. blood pressure.
   B. pulse rate.
   C. level of pain.
   D. mental status.
   E. both A and B.

MATCHING

Write the letter of the term in the space provided next to the appropriate description.

A. epistaxis

B. varicosities

C. sick sinus syndrome

D. autonomic dysfunction

E. transient ischemic attack

F. brain ischemia

G. urosepsis

H. nocturia

I. polycythemia

J. delirium

K. senile dementia

L. vertigo

M. mesenteric infarct

N. spondylosis

O. dysphoria

©2013 Pearson Education, Inc.
Paramedic Care: Principles & Practice, Vol. 6, 4th Ed.

_____ 81. Acute alteration in mental functioning that is often reversible

_____ 82. Septicemia originating from the urinary tract

_____ 83. Medical term for a nosebleed

_____ 84. Excessive urination, usually at night

_____ 85. Death of tissue in the peritoneal fold that encircles the small intestine

_____ 86. Exaggerated feeling of depression or unrest

_____ 87. Excess of red blood cells

_____ 88. Abnormal dilation of a vein

_____ 89. Group of disorders characterized by dysfunction of the sinoatrial node

_____ 90. Sensation of faintness or dizziness causing loss of balance

_____ 91. General term used to describe an abnormal decline in mental function in the elderly

_____ 92. Degeneration of the vertebral body

_____ 93. Abnormality of the involuntary aspect of the nervous system

_____ 94. Injury to the brain tissues caused by an inadequate supply of oxygen and nutrients

_____ 95. Medical condition similar to a stroke but reversible and commonly involving syncope

Special Project

Common Age-Related Systemic Changes

Complete the chart on this page, showing the systemic changes that come with age and the clinical importance of these changes.

Body System	Changes with Age	Clinical Importance
Respiratory		
Cardiovascular		
Neurological		
Endocrine		
Gastrointestinal		
Thermoregulatory		
Integumentary (Skin)		
Musculoskeletal		
Renal		
Genitourinary		
Immune		
Hematological		

Abuse, Neglect, and Assault

Review of Chapter Objectives

In each chapter of the workbook, we identify the objectives and the important elements of the text content. You should review these items and refer to the pages listed if any points are not clear.

After reading this chapter, you should be able to:

1. Define key terms introduced in this chapter.   **p. 182**

Knowing and being able to apply the key terms in each chapter is critical to understanding chapter concepts. Write the list of key terms. Then write the definition of each one in your own words. Check your understanding by confirming the definitions in the text glossary. Correct any misunderstandings. Create a study aid by writing each key term on the front of an index card and the definition on the back. Use the cards to quiz yourself, or to have someone quiz you.

2. Describe the epidemiology and demographics of abuse, assault, and neglect.   **p. 183**

Because of underreporting, it is difficult to provide accurate statistics on the incidence of abuse and assault in the United States today. That makes available figures even more overwhelming in their seriousness. To grasp the magnitude of the problem, consider these facts:

- Nearly 3 million children suffer abuse each year and almost five children a day die as a result of child abuse.
- Between 2 and 4 million women each year are battered by their partners or spouses.
- Elder abuse occurs at an incidence of 700,000 to 1.1 million annually.

3. Describe the characteristics of abusers and abused and neglected patients, including partner abuse, elder abuse, and child abuse.   **pp. 184–187**

Characteristics of Partner Abusers

Partner abuse occurs in all demographic groups. However, abuse is more common in lower socioeconomic levels in which wage earners have trouble paying bills, holding down jobs, or keeping pace with technological changes. Typically the abuser does not like being out of control but at the same time feels powerless to change. A spouse or partner abuser usually exhibits an overly aggressive personality—an outgrowth of low self-esteem. They often feel insecure and jealous, flying into sudden and unpredictable rages. Use of alcohol or drugs increases the likelihood that the abuser will lose control and may not even remember his actions.

In the aftermath of an abusive incident, the abuser often feels a sense of remorse and shame. The person may seek to relieve his guilt by promising to change or even seeking help. For a time, the abuser may appear charming or loving, convincing an abused spouse or partner to think the pattern has finally been broken. All too often, however, the cycle of violence repeats itself in just a few days, weeks, or months.

Characteristics of Abused Elders

Like partner abuse, elder abuse cuts across all demographic groups. As a result, it is difficult to profile the people who are most likely to abuse elders. However, several characteristics are found in abusers of the elderly. Often, the perpetrators exhibit alcoholic behavior, drug addiction, or some mental impairment. The abuser may also be dependent upon the income or assistance of the elder—a situation that can cause resentment, anger, and, in some cases, violence. According to one study, in cases of domestic elder abuse, the most typical abusers are adult children who are overstressed by care of the elder and/or who were abused themselves.

Characteristics of Child Abusers

As with other types of abusers, you cannot relate child abuse to social class, income, or education. However, most child abusers share one common trait: They were physically or emotionally abused as children. They often would prefer to use other forms of discipline, but under stress they regress to their earliest and most familiar patterns. Once they have resorted to physical discipline, the punishments become more severe and more frequent.

In cases of reported physical abuse, perpetrators tend to be men. However, the statistics for men and women even out when neglect is taken into account. Although potential child abusers can include a wide variety of caregivers, one or both parents are the most likely abusers. Frequent behavioral traits include use or abuse of alcohol and/or drugs, immaturity, self-absorption, and an inability to emotionally identify with the child.

Characteristics of Sexual Assailants

Once again, sexual assailants can come from almost any background. However, the violent victimizers of children are substantially more likely than the victimizers of adults to have been physically or sexually abused as children. Many assailants, particularly adolescents and abusive adults, think domination is part of any relationship. Such thinking can lead to date rape or marital rape. In a significant number of all cases, the assailants are under the influence of alcohol or drugs.

4. **Adapt your approach to history and assessment to interact effectively with abused or neglected patients.**   **pp. 191–192**

Your primary responsibility on a call involving an abusive situation is safety—both your own and that of the patient. You should never enter a scene if your safety is compromised, and you should leave the scene as soon as you feel unsafe.

You can expect the victims of abuse to feel threatened as a result of the violence they have suffered. One of your main duties is to provide a safe environment for an already traumatized patient. Sometimes you can provide safety merely by your official presence. Other times, you may have to move the patient to the ambulance so you can relocate to a different environment. In still other situations, you may have to summon additional personnel, such as law enforcement.

Specific assessment and management considerations will depend upon the type of abuse encountered. In cases of partner abuse, use direct questions, if possible, to convey an awareness that the person's partner may have contributed to the injury. In cases of suspected child abuse, examine the patient for identifiable patterns of physical mistreatment or neglect and record your objective observations. In cases of sexual abuse, use open-ended questions to reestablish a sense of control. If possible, allow a same-sex crew member to maintain contact with the victim.

Regardless of the situation, keep in mind that the patient has been harmed by another human being, in many cases a person that he or she knows intimately. Try to transport the patient to the hospital. If

©2013 Pearson Education, Inc.
Paramedic Care: Principles & Practice, Vol. 6, 4th Ed.

you cannot do so, either because of patient refusal or intervention by the suspected abuser, be sure to report your suspicions to the appropriate authorities or agencies.

5. Explain the importance of communicating the availability of resources to patients in suspected partner abuse situations. p. 191

Specialized resources include both private and state or federally funded programs. Make a point of learning about hospital units for the victims of sexual assault, public and private shelters for battered persons, and state agencies responsible for youth and their families.

Also acquaint yourself with nurses trained as sexual assault nurse examiners (SANEs). They have completed programs allowing them to perform the physical exam for sexual assaults.

6. Explain the ethical and legal obligations to report suspected abuse and neglect. p. 191

Abuse and assault constitute crimes. Although their nature and the extent of the crime often depend upon local laws, you have a responsibility to report suspected cases. Because the assailants may be detained only a short time, you also have an obligation to find out about the victim and witness protection programs available in your area.

Study the local laws and protocols regarding cases of abuse and assault. All 50 states require health care workers to report suspected cases of child abuse. Some states require EMS personnel to report even a suspicion of abuse or assault. Some states allow minors to seek medical care for sexual assault without parental consent. The Joint Commission mandates that hospital personnel screen incoming patients for abuse. Regardless of where you live, take time to learn the rules and regulations that affect your practice, both for your sake and for the sake of your patient.

7. Identify patterns of injuries and behavior suspicious for abuse and neglect. pp. 184; 186; 187–189; 190

Examples of Spouse/Partner Abuse
Partner abuse can fall into several categories. The most obvious form is physical abuse, which involves the application of force in ways too numerous to list. In addition to direct injury, physical abuse may exacerbate existing medical conditions, such as hypertension, diabetes, or asthma. Verbal abuse, which consists of words chosen to control or harm a person, may leave no physical mark. However, it damages a person's self-esteem and can lead to depression, substance abuse, or other self-destructive behavior. As noted in objective 2, partner abuse can also take the form of sexual abuse—unwanted, forced sexual contact between two people.

Examples of Elder Abuse
Elder abuse can also be physical, verbal, or sexual. In some cases, signs of elder abuse are subtle, such as theft of the victim's belongings or loss of freedom. Other signs, such as wounds, untreated decubitus ulcers, or poor hygiene, are more obvious.

Examples of Child Abuse
Children very commonly get injured, and not all injured children are abused. Conditions commonly mistaken for abuse are car seat burns, staphylococcal scalded skin syndrome, chickenpox (cigarette burns), and hematological disorders that can cause bruising. In assessing a child, look for common patterns of physical abuse, evidence of emotional abuse, and/or environmental clues of neglect.

Children can be shaken, thrown, burned or scalded, and battered with almost any kind of object. They can be denied food, clean clothing, medical care, or even access to a toilet. The damage done to a child can last a lifetime and perpetuate a cycle of violence for generations to come.

Examples of Sexual Abuse/Assault
Sexual abuse/assault typically involves a male assailant and a female victim, but not always. Forced sexual contact can range from exposure to fondling to rape to sexual torture. Sexual assault and rape carry serious consequences. Victims may be physically injured, or even killed, during the assault. They commonly suffer internal injuries, particularly if multiple assailants are involved in the attack. Rape can

result in infections, sexually transmitted diseases, and unwanted pregnancies. The psychological damage is deep and long lasting. Shame, anger, and a lack of trust can persist for years—or even for a lifetime.

8. Describe special considerations in interacting with victims of sexual assault. pp. 190–192

You can expect victims of assault or abuse to feel unsafe as a result of the violence they have suffered. One of your primary responsibilities is to provide a safe environment for an already traumatized patient. Sometimes you can provide safety merely by your official presence. Other times, you may have to move the patient to the ambulance, where you can lock the doors, or move to a different location entirely. In still other instances, you may have to summon additional personnel.

You are also responsible for providing proper psychosocial care for the victims of abuse and assault. Privacy is a major consideration. In many cases, a paramedic of the same sex as the victim should maintain contact with the victim. Although you may need to expose the victim during assessment, you should cover the patient and remove him or her from public view as soon as possible.

When talking with the patient, use open-ended questions to reestablish a sense of control. Remain nonjudgmental throughout treatment, avoiding subjective comments about both the patient and the assailant. In a reassuring voice, encourage the patient to report the rape, explaining the importance of preserving evidence.

Medical treatment of victims of abuse and assault is essentially the same as with other patients. However, you should always remember the origins of the patient's injuries and provide appropriate emotional support. Keep in mind that the patient has been harmed by another human being, in many cases a person that the patient knows intimately.

9. Recognize the effects of date rape drugs. pp. 190–191

The use of drugs to facilitate a sexual assault is occurring with increasing frequency. These medications will generally render a person unresponsive or weaken the person to the point of being unable to resist an attacker. Some of these medications cause amnesia, thus eliminating or distorting the victim's recall of the assault. Because these drugs have become more commonplace in society, it is important for EMS personnel to be aware of these agents and their effects. Date rape drugs have a rapid onset of action with a varying duration of effect. Drugs that have been associated with rape, which are also known as predator drugs, include the following:

- **Rohypnol.** Rohypnol is a potent benzodiazepine that produces a sedative effect, amnesia, muscle relaxation, and slowing of the psychomotor response. It is widely prescribed outside the United States as a sleeping pill. It is colorless, odorless, and tasteless and can be dissolved in a drink without being detected. Rohypnol can be potentiated by the concomitant effects of alcohol. Street names for rohypnol include Roofies, Rope, Ruffies, R2, Ruffles, Roche, Forget-Pill, and Mexican Valium.
- **GHB.** Gamma-hydroxybutyrate, commonly called GHB, is an odorless, colorless liquid depressant with anesthetic-type qualities. It is also used as an amino acid supplement by body builders. The drug causes relaxation, tranquility, sensuality, and loss of inhibitions. Street names for GHB include Liquid Ecstasy, Liquid X, Scoop, Easy Lay, and Grievous Bodily Harm.
- **Ketamine.** Ketamine is a potent anesthetic agent. Widely used in veterinary practice, ketamine is also used in human anesthesia. It is chemically similar to the hallucinogenic LSD. It causes hallucinations, amnesia, and dissociation. Street names for ketamine include K, Special K, Vitamin K, Jet, and Super Acid.
- **MDMA.** 3,4-Methylenedioxymethamphetamine (MDMA) is most commonly known as Ecstasy. It is known to cause psychological difficulties including confusion, depression, sleep problems, drug craving, severe anxiety, and paranoia (both during and sometimes weeks after taking the drug). It can also cause physical symptoms such as muscle tension, involuntary teeth clenching, nausea, blurred vision, rapid eye movement, faintness, and chills or sweating. Street names for MDMA, in addition to Ecstasy, include Beans, Adam, XTC, Roll, E, and M.

10. Describe the epidemiology of hate crimes. p. 192

A hate crime is a crime of hatred or prejudice in which the perpetrator targets a particular victim or victims because of the victim's perceived membership in a certain social group. These groups can

©2013 Pearson Education, Inc.
Paramedic Care: Principles & Practice, Vol. 6, 4th Ed.

include racial, religious, sexual orientation, political, disability, and other social groups. The crime is based on bias and sometimes referred to as bias-motivated crime. Most hate crimes result from racial bias. This is followed by religious bias, sexual orientation bias, ethnicity/national origin bias, and disability bias. The vast majority of racial hate crimes are against blacks. Most religious hate crimes are directed at Jews. In terms of sexual orientation bias, most hate crimes are motivated by anti-male homosexual bias. Anti-female homosexual hate crimes are much less common. Most ethnicity/national origin hate crimes are directed at Hispanics.

Most hate crimes involve vandalism. Intimidation is also common. Approximately one in three hate crimes involves assault. Certain hate crimes, especially those that are racially motivated, can result in widespread violence. EMS can become involved in any aspect of hate crimes, from simple intimidation to full-fledged riots. Paramedics must recognize that hate crimes and their aftermath are emotionally charged events and paramedics, because of their race, gender, or sexual orientation, can be drawn into the fray. Always treat hate crimes as particularly dangerous situations. Involve law enforcement early and always ensure the safety of you and your partner first.

11. **Document relevant observations and information regarding suspected abuse, neglect, hate crimes, and sexual assault.** pp. 183–192

It is important that you carefully and objectively document all your findings. Your actions can affect the outcome of a case or prosecution of a crime. If the patient tells you something about the abuser or assailant, mark it with quotation marks on the patient care report. In the case of rape, patients should not urinate, defecate, douche, bathe, eat, drink, or smoke. Some jurisdictions have specific rules for evidence protection, such as using paper bags to collect evidence or placing bags over the patient's hands to preserve trace evidence. Remember that any evidence you collect must remain in your custody until you can give it directly to a law enforcement official to preserve the chain of evidence. Regardless of the emotions evoked by the call, when documenting the incident, you must be completely factual and nonjudgmental.

Case Study Review

Reread the case study on page 183 in Paramedic Care: Special Patients; *then, read the following discussion.*

The case study draws attention to the role of the paramedic on a call involving a female victim of sexual assault. It highlights the importance of emotional support for the victim and the legal ramifications of any documentation, particularly the narrative.

Fortunately, the patient in this case experienced no life-threatening injuries. Unfortunately, she has been psychologically scarred—perhaps for life—by this horrifying incident. Deciding to use the female crew member to conduct the assessment and most of the management was a wise decision. However, if a female crew member was unavailable, whoever cared for the patient should exhibit a compassionate and consoling attitude. The presence of a police officer ensured scene safety, but if the patient still felt vulnerable, it would have been appropriate (upon discussion with law enforcement) to move her to the ambulance.

It was important for the crew to examine the patient carefully, while protecting her privacy as well as any evidence. Although it was not specifically stated in the case, it is essential to use nonjudgmental language and to remain conscious of all body language. In such instances, you should ask open-ended questions, encouraging the patient to talk and to regain a sense of control. Limiting unnecessary involvement by EMS responders would also be helpful for the patient. You may want to ask the patient who should be called or informed of the incident.

Your actions toward a victim of abuse or assault can help begin the long road to psychological recovery. Furthermore, as pointed out in the case, your response may impact on the outcome of a case if you are called to testify at a later time.

Content Self-Evaluation

MULTIPLE CHOICE

_____ 1. Partner abuse is defined as physical or emotional violence from a man or woman toward a co-worker.
  A. True
  B. False

_____ 2. The most widespread and best-known form of abuse involves the abuse of
  A. women by men.
  B. children by their mothers.
  C. children by their fathers.
  D. elders by their children.
  E. same-sex partners.

_____ 3. Many victims of abuse hesitate or fail to report the problem because of a
  A. fear of reprisal.
  B. lack of knowledge.
  C. fear of humiliation.
  D. lack of financial resources.
  E. all of the above.

_____ 4. By far the most common characteristic of abusers—whether they be partner abusers, child abusers, or elder abusers—is a
  A. history of substance abuse.
  B. lack of employment.
  C. family history of violence.
  D. lack of education.
  E. mental impairment.

_____ 5. Forty-five percent of pregnant women suffer some form of battery during pregnancy.
  A. True
  B. False

_____ 6. In assessing the battered patient, all of the following are appropriate actions, EXCEPT
  A. direct questioning.
  B. asking the victim why she or he doesn't leave.
  C. rehearsing the quickest way to leave the home.
  D. nonjudgmental questioning.
  E. reminding the patient that assault is a crime.

_____ 7. All of the following are causes of elder abuse, EXCEPT
  A. stress on middle-aged caregivers.
  B. decreased life expectancies.
  C. physical and mental impairments.
  D. limited resources for long-term care.
  E. decreased productivity in later years.

_____ 8. Which of the following are two main types of elder abuse?
  A. Neglect and domestic
  B. Emotional and financial
  C. Domestic and institutional
  D. Mental and institutional
  E. Financial and domestic

_____ 9. The perpetrators of domestic elder abuse tend to be
  A. paid caregivers.
  B. siblings.
  C. adult children.
  D. spouses.
  E. friends or neighbors.

_____ 10. In cases of child abuse, the most likely abusers are
  A. babysitters.
  B. siblings.
  C. strangers.
  D. one or both parents.
  E. friends charged with the child's care.

©2013 Pearson Education, Inc.
Paramedic Care: Principles & Practice, Vol. 6, 4th Ed.

11. All of the following are characteristics of abused children, EXCEPT
A. sudden behavioral changes.
B. neediness.
C. absence of nearly all emotion.
D. unusual wariness.
E. concern over a parent's absence.

12. One of the signs of intentional scalding of a child is
A. staphylococcal scalded skin.
B. hematological disorders.
C. multiple splatter marks.
D. multiple bruises.
E. absence of splash burns.

13. Children rarely exhibit accidental fractures to the
A. head.
B. ribs.
C. legs.
D. arms.
E. hands or feet.

14. Which type of injury claims the largest number of lives among abused children?
A. Malnutrition
B. Head injuries
C. Burns
D. Chest injury
E. Abdominal injuries

15. The group most likely to be victims of sexual assault or rape are adolescent females under age 18.
A. True
B. False

16. The victims of rape most commonly describe their assailant as a stranger.
A. True
B. False

17. When talking to a rape victim, you can help the patient regain a sense of self-control by asking
A. open-ended questions.
B. closed-ended questions.
C. indirect questions.
D. nonpersonal questions.
E. leading questions.

18. Sexual assault nurse examiners (SANEs) are specially trained health care workers who can
A. help with the prehospital care report.
B. protect the patient against the assailant.
C. provide information on the protection of evidence.
D. protect EMS crews against legal suits.
E. none of the above.

19. In managing a rape case, honor the patient's request to bathe or shower.
A. True
B. False

20. All 50 states require health care workers to report suspected cases of
A. child abuse.
B. rape.
C. elder abuse.
D. spousal abuse.
E. partner abuse.

MATCHING

Write the letter of the term in the space provided next to the appropriate description.

A. partner abuse

B. sexual assault

C. rape

D. institutional elder abuse

E. hate crime

F. domestic elder abuse

G. SANE

H. chain of evidence

I. battered

J. child abuse

_____ **21.** Patients who have been physically struck by an abuser

_____ **22.** Crime of hatred or prejudice in which the perpetrator targets a particular victim or victims because of the victim's perceived membership in a certain social group

_____ **23.** Physical or emotional violence or neglect when an elder is being cared for in a home-based setting

_____ **24.** Penile penetration of the genitalia without the consent of the victim

_____ **25.** Physical or emotional violence or neglect toward a person from infancy to 18 years of age

_____ **26.** Physical or emotional violence or neglect when an elder is being cared for by a person paid to provide care

_____ **27.** Legally retaining and knowing the whereabouts of items pertinent to a rape or assault

_____ **28.** Nurse specially trained to examine the victims of sexual assault

_____ **29.** Physical or emotional violence toward a wife, husband, date, or live-in companion

_____ **30.** Unwanted oral, genital, or manual sexual contact

Special Project

Breaking the Cycle of Abuse: Support Services

Having the telephone numbers of the abuse hotlines and referral services within your state, region, or community can help the victim or the abuser take steps toward breaking the cycle of abuse before it is repeated or passed on to another generation. Take the time to investigate the contact numbers and the resources/services that can be provided for each of the following in your area:

DOMESTIC VIOLENCE		
Name of agency	Contact number	Services provided

CHILD ABUSE		
Name of agency	Contact number	Services provided

ELDER ABUSE		
Name of agency	Contact number	Services provided

SEXUAL ABUSE		
Name of agency	Contact number	Services provided

Now take one more step. Make a copy of this information and carry it onboard the ambulance or write the phone numbers into the pocket reference that you carry in your uniform pocket!

The Challenged Patient

Review of Chapter Objectives

In each chapter of the workbook, we identify the objectives and the important elements of the text content. You should review these items and refer to the pages listed if any points are not clear.

After reading this chapter, you should be able to:

1. **Define key terms introduced in this chapter.** **p. 196**

   Knowing and being able to apply the key terms in each chapter is critical to understanding chapter concepts. Write the list of key terms. Then write the definition of each one in your own words. Check your understanding by confirming the definitions in the text glossary. Correct any misunderstandings. Create a study aid by writing each key term on the front of an index card and the definition on the back. Use the cards to quiz yourself, or to have someone quiz you.

2. **Describe the epidemiology and demographics of each of the following challenges:**

   a. **Vision impairment** **pp. 198–199**
   When caring for the patient with a visual impairment, it is important to note whether the impairment is a permanent disability or a new symptom as a result of the illness or injury for which you were called. It is necessary to understand the causes of blindness before this determination can be made. Visual impairments can result from a number of causes, including injury, disease, congenital conditions, infection (such as cytomegalovirus [CMV]), and degeneration of the retina, optic nerve, or nerve pathways.

   b. **Hearing impairment** **pp. 197–198**
   Hearing impairments involve a decrease or loss in the ability to distinguish or hear sounds, particularly those involving speech. An inability to hear is commonly described as deafness. A person may be completely deaf or partially deaf. A person may be deaf in one ear or both ears. The condition may be present at birth or may occur later in life as a result of an accident, illness, or aging.

   The two basic types of deafness are conductive deafness and sensorineural deafness. Conductive deafness results from any condition that prevents sound waves from being transmitted from the external ear to the middle or inner ear. The condition can be either temporary or permanent. Sensorineural deafness arises from the inability of nerve impulses to reach the auditory center of the brain because of damage either to the inner ear or to the brain itself. It is usually a permanent condition.

Other causes might be the temporary blockage of the ear canal by various irritants, such as dust, hair spray, insects, or water ("swimmer's ear"). Patient attempts to clean the canal with cotton applicators may disrupt the ear's natural cleaning process and push the debris deeper into the ear, which sets the stage for bacterial infections and conductive deafness. Obstructions can also be caused by hematomas, which may result from blunt trauma to the ear.

c. **Speech impairment**   pp. 199–200

You may encounter four types of speech impairment: language disorders, articulation disorders, voice production disorders, and fluency disorders.

A language disorder is an impaired ability to understand the spoken or written word. The loss of the ability to communicate in speech, writing, or signs is known as aphasia. Aphasia can manifest itself as sensory aphasia, in which a person can no longer understand the spoken word; motor aphasia, in which a person can no longer use the symbols of speech; and global aphasia, in which a person has both sensory and motor aphasia.

Articulation disorders, also known as dysarthria, affect the way a person's speech is heard by others. When a patient has a voice production disorder, the quality of the person's voice is affected. This can be caused by trauma or may be due to overuse of the vocal cords or infection. Cancer of the larynx can also cause a speech failure by impeding air from passing through the vocal cords. Fluency disorders present as stuttering. Although the cause of stuttering is not fully understood, the condition is found more often in men than in women. Stuttering occurs when sounds or syllables are repeated and the patient cannot put words together fluidly.

d. **Obesity**   pp. 200–201

More than 40 percent of people in the United States are considered obese, and many more are heavier than their ideal body weight. Besides the obvious difficulty of lifting and moving the obese patient, excess weight can exacerbate the complaint for which you were called. Obesity can also lead to a number of serious medical conditions, including hypertension, heart disease, strokes, diabetes, and joint and muscle problems.

People require a certain amount of body fat to metabolize vitamins and minerals. Obesity occurs when a person has an abnormal amount of body fat and a weight 20 to 30 percent heavier than is normal for people of the same age, gender, and height. Morbid obesity is defined as a person who is 50 to 100 percent, or 100 pounds, above his ideal body weight. Morbidly obese persons are at increased risk for diabetes, hypertension, heart disease, stroke, certain cancers (breast and colon), depression, and osteoarthritis.

Obesity occurs for a number of reasons. In many cases, it happens when a person's caloric intake is higher than the amount of calories required to meet his energy needs. In such cases, diet, exercise, and lifestyle choices play a role in the person's condition. Genetic factors may also predispose a patient toward obesity. In rare cases, an obese patient may have a low basal metabolic rate, which causes the body to burn calories at a slower rate. In such cases, the condition may be produced by an illness, particularly hypothyroidism.

e. **Paralysis**   p. 202

A paralyzed patient may be paraplegic or quadriplegic. A paraplegic patient has been paralyzed from the waist down; a quadriplegic patient has paralysis of all four extremities. In addition, spinal cord injuries in the area of C3 to C5 and above may also paralyze the patient's respiratory muscles and compromise the ability to breathe. If your patient depends on a home ventilator, it is important to maintain a patent airway and to keep the ventilator functioning. Also, a paralyzed patient may have been breathing through a tracheostomy for some time. If the patient has suffered a recent spinal cord injury, halo traction may still be intact.

f. **Mental illness**   p. 202

Mental and emotional illnesses may range from psychoses such as schizophrenia to personality disorders to psychological conditions resulting from trauma. Emotional impairments can include such conditions as anxiety or depression. For a detailed discussion of the etiologies, assessment, management, and treatment of these patients, see Volume 4, Chapter 11.

g. **Developmental disabilities**   pp. 202–203

People with developmental disabilities are individuals with impaired or insufficient development of the brain who are unable to learn at the usual rate. In recent years, large numbers of people with developmental disabilities have been mainstreamed into the day-to-day activities of life. They hold jobs and live in residential settings, either on their own, with their families, or in group homes.

©2013 Pearson Education, Inc.
Paramedic Care: Principles & Practice, Vol. 6, 4th Ed.

Developmental disabilities can have a variety of causes. They can be genetic, such as in Down syndrome, or they can be the product of brain injury caused by some hypoxic or traumatic event. Such injuries can take place before birth, during birth, or anytime thereafter.

h. Emotional disabilities   p. 207

Caring for a terminally ill patient is an emotional challenge. Many times, the patient will choose to die at home, but at the last minute the family will compromise those wishes by calling for an ambulance. In other cases, the patient may call for an ambulance so that a newly developed condition can be treated or a medication adjusted. For more on caring for the terminally ill, either at home or in a hospice situation, see Chapter 8 in this volume.

i. Cognitive disabilities (such as those associated with past traumatic brain injury)   p. 206

A patient with a previous head injury may not be recognized easily. You may not notice anything different about the patient until the person starts to speak. A patient who has had a head injury may display symptoms similar to those of a stroke, without the hemiparesis, or paralysis, to one side of the body. The presenting symptoms will be related to the area of the brain that has been injured. The patient may have aphasia, slurred speech, loss of vision or hearing, or a learning disability. Such patients may also exhibit short-term memory loss and may not have any recollection of their original injury.

j. Physical disabilities (such arthritis and neuromuscular and movement disorders)   pp. 203–207

Arthritis. The three most common types of arthritis are juvenile rheumatoid arthritis (JRA), a connective tissue disorder that strikes before age 16; rheumatoid arthritis, an autoimmune disorder; and osteoarthritis, a degenerative joint disease, the most common arthritis seen in elderly patients. All forms of arthritis cause painful swelling and irritation of the joints, making everyday tasks sometimes impossible. Arthritis patients commonly have joint stiffness and limited range of motion. Sometimes the smaller joints of the hands and feet become deformed. In addition, children with JRA may suffer complications involving the spleen or liver.

Cerebral Palsy. Cerebral palsy is a group of disorders caused by damage to the cerebrum in utero or by trauma during birth. Prenatal exposure of the mother to German measles can cause cerebral palsy, along with any event that leads to hypoxia in the fetus. Premature birth or brain damage from a difficult delivery can also lead to cerebral palsy. Other causes include encephalitis, meningitis, or head injury from a fall or the abuse of an infant.

Patients with cerebral palsy have difficulty controlling motor functions, causing spasticity of the muscles. This condition may affect a single limb or the entire body. About two-thirds of cerebral palsy patients have a below-normal intellectual capacity, and about half experience seizures. Conversely, a full third of patients with cerebral palsy have normal intelligence and a few are highly gifted.

The three main types of cerebral palsy are spastic paralysis, athetosis, and ataxia. Spastic paralysis, which is the most common form of cerebral palsy, forces the muscles into a state of permanent stiffness and contracture. When both legs are affected, the knees turn inward, causing the characteristic "scissor gait." Athetosis causes an involuntary writhing movement, usually affecting arms, feet, hands, and legs. If the patient's face is affected, the person may demonstrate drooling or grimacing. Ataxic cerebral palsy is the rarest form of the disease and causes problems with coordination of gait and balance.

Multiple Sclerosis. Multiple sclerosis (MS) is a disorder of the central nervous system that usually strikes between the ages of 20 and 40, affecting women more often than men. The exact cause of MS is unknown, but it is considered to be an autoimmune disorder. Characteristically, repeated inflammation of the myelin sheath surrounding the nerves leads to scar tissue, which in turn blocks nerve impulses to the affected area.

The onset of MS is slow. It starts with a slight change in the strength of a muscle and a numbness or tingling in the affected muscle. Doctors encourage patients with MS to lead as normal a life as possible, but they become increasingly tired. Their gait may become unsteady, and they may slur their speech. Patients with MS may also develop eye problems, such as double vision, owing to weakness of the eye muscles, or eye pain due to neuritis of the optic nerve.

Muscular Dystrophy. Muscular dystrophy (MD) is a group of hereditary disorders characterized by progressive weakness and wasting of muscle tissue. It is a genetic disorder, leading to gradual degeneration of muscle fibers. The most common form of MD is Duchenne muscular dystrophy, which typically affects boys between the ages of 3 and 6. It leads to progressive muscle weakness in the legs and pelvis and to paralysis by age 12. Ultimately, the disease affects the respiratory muscles and heart, causing death at an early age. The other various MD disorders are classified by the age of the patient at onset of symptoms and by the muscles affected.

Poliomyelitis. Poliomyelitis, commonly called polio, is a communicable disease that affects the gray matter of the brain and the spinal cord. Although it is highly contagious, immunization has made outbreaks of polio extremely rare in developed nations. However, it is important to know about polio because many people born before development of the polio vaccination in the 1950s have been affected by the disease.

Typically, the polio virus enters the body through the gastrointestinal tract. It circulates through the digestive tract and then enters the bloodstream. There, it is carried to the central nervous system, where the virus enters and alters the nerve cells. In cases of paralytic poliomyelitis, patients experience asymmetrical muscle weakness that leads to permanent paralysis.

Although most patients recover from the disease itself, they are left with permanent paralysis of the affected muscles. You may recognize a polio victim by the use of assistive devices for ambulation or by the reduced size of the affected limb, which is a result of muscle atrophy. Some patients may have experienced paralysis of the respiratory muscles and require assisted ventilation. Patients on long-term ventilators will typically have tracheostomies.

A related disorder is called post-polio syndrome. Post-polio syndrome can develop in patients who suffered severely from polio more than 30 years ago. Although the cause of post-polio syndrome remains unknown, researchers think the condition results from the stress of long-term weakness in the affected nerves. Patients with this condition tire quickly, especially after exercise, and develop an intolerance for cold in their extremities. Unfortunately, some persons who survived their original bout with polio die in later years from the effects of post-polio syndrome.

Spina Bifida. Spina bifida is a congenital abnormality that falls under the category of neural tube defects. It presents when there is a defect in the closure of the backbone and the spinal canal. In spina bifida occulta, the patient exhibits few outward signs of the deformity. In spina bifida cystica, the failure of the closure allows the spinal cord and covering membranes to protrude from the back, causing an obvious deformity.

Myasthenia Gravis. Myasthenia gravis is an autoimmune disease characterized by chronic weakness of voluntary muscles and progressive fatigue. The condition results from a problem with the neurotransmitters, which causes a blocking of nerve signals to the muscles. It occurs most frequently in women between the ages of 20 and 50.

k. Chronic and terminal illnesses (such as cancer, cystic fibrosis, and communicable illnesses) pp. 204–205; 207–208

Cancer. Cancer is really a blanket term for many different diseases, each with its own characteristics but having in common the abnormal growth of cells in normal tissue. The primary site of origin of the cancer cells determines the type of cancer that the patient has. If the cancer starts in epithelial tissue, it is called a carcinoma. If the cancer forms in connective tissue, it is called a sarcoma.

It may be difficult for you to recognize a cancer patient, because the disease often has few obvious signs and symptoms. However, treatments for the disease do tend to produce telltale signs, such as alopecia (hair loss) or anorexia (loss of appetite) leading to weight loss. Tattoos may be left on the skin by radiation oncologists to mark positioning of radiation therapy equipment. In addition, physical changes, such as removal of a breast (mastectomy), may be obvious.

If patients have recently undergone chemotherapy, assume that they are neutropenic. Reduce their exposure to infection as much as possible. Remember that, once infected, a neutropenic patient can quickly go into septic shock, sometimes in a matter of hours.

Also keep in mind that cancer patients' veins may have become scarred and difficult to access as a result of frequent IV starts, blood draws, and caustic chemotherapy transfusions. A patient with cancer may also have an implanted infusion port, found just below the skin, with the catheter inserted into the subclavian vein or brachial artery. Patients with cancer may also have a peripheral access device, such as a Groshong catheter or Hickman catheter, which has access ports that extend outside the skin.

©2013 Pearson Education, Inc.
Paramedic Care: Principles & Practice, Vol. 6, 4th Ed.

Cystic Fibrosis. Cystic fibrosis (CF or mucoviscidosis) is an inherited disorder that involves the exocrine (mucus-producing) glands, primarily in the lungs and the digestive system. Thick mucus forms in the lungs, causing bronchial obstruction and atelectasis, or collapse of the alveoli. In addition, the thick mucus causes blockages in the small ducts of the pancreas, leading to a decrease in the pancreatic enzymes needed for digestion. This results in malnutrition, even for patients on healthy diets.

A unique characteristic of CF is the high concentration of chloride in the sweat, leading to the use of a diagnostic test known as the "sweat test." A patient with CF may also suffer from frequent lung infections, clay-colored stools, or clubbing of the fingers or toes.

Recent medical advances have extended the lives of patients with CF so that some live well into their 30s. However, because of a poor prognosis, most of the patients with CF whom you see will be children and adolescents.

Communicable Diseases. When treating people with communicable diseases, you should withhold all personal judgment. Although you will have to take Standard Precautions just as you would with any patient, keep in mind the heightened sensitivity of a person with a communicable disease. Most of these patients are familiar with the health care setting and understand why you must take certain protective measures. However, you should still explain that you take these measures with all patients that have similar diseases. Also, you do not need to take additional precautions that are not required by departmental policy. The patient will generally spot these extra measures and feel guilt, shame, or anger.

3. **Adapt your approach to communication, history taking, assessment, and management to interact effectively with patients with a variety of pathologic problems and sensory, physical, mental, emotional, cognitive, and developmental disabilities.**   pp. 197–208

Hearing impairments. It is important to detect deafness early in your assessment. A partially deaf person may ask questions repeatedly, misunderstand answers to questions, or respond inappropriately. Such reactions can easily be mistaken for head injury, leading to misdirected treatment. The most obvious sign of deafness is a hearing aid. Unfortunately, hearing aids do not work for all types of deafness. Also, many people do not wear hearing aids, even when they have been prescribed. In addition, deaf people may have poor diction due to partial hearing loss or hearing loss later in life. They might use their hands to gesture or use sign language. As noted, deaf people may ask you to speak louder or they may speak excessively loudly themselves. Finally, deaf people will commonly face you so that they can read your lips.

When managing a patient with a hearing impairment, you can do several things to ease communication. Begin by identifying yourself and making sure the patient knows that you are speaking to him. Get the patient's attention by moving so you can be seen or by gently touching the person, if appropriate. By addressing deaf patients face to face, you give them the opportunity to read your lips and interpret your expression.

When talking with a deaf patient, speak slowly in a normal voice. Don't forget one of the most simple and effective means of communication: use of pen and paper. Finally, many people with hearing impairments know sign language, usually American Sign Language (ASL). If you do not know sign language, try to find an interpreter, such as a family member or even a neighbor.

Visual Impairments. Depending on the degree of impairment and a person's adjustment to the loss of vision, you may or may not recognize the condition right away. In cases of obvious blindness, identify yourself as you approach the patient so the person knows you are there. Also, describe everything you are doing as you do it.

Many people who are blind have tools to assist them in their activities of daily living. The most obvious is a service dog. When approaching a person with a service dog, do not pet the dog or disturb it while the dog is in its harness. For the dog, the harness means that it is working. Ask permission from the patient to touch the dog. Never grab the leash, the harness, or the patient's arm without asking permission. Doing this may place you, the dog, or the owner in danger. Accommodation must be made for transporting the guide dog with the patient. Circumstances and local protocols will dictate whether you transport the dog in the ambulance with the patient or have the dog transported in another vehicle.

If your patient does not have a guide dog, inquire about other tools that the person may want brought to the hospital. If the patient is ambulatory, have the person take your arm for guidance rather than taking the patient's arm.

Speech Impairments. When speaking to a patient with a speech impairment, never assume that the person lacks intelligence. It will be difficult, if not impossible, to complete a thorough interview if you have insulted the patient. Do not to rush the patient or predict an answer. Try to form questions that require short, direct answers. Prepare to spend extra time during your interview.

When asking questions, look directly at the patient. If you cannot understand what the person has said, politely ask him to repeat it. Never pretend to understand when you don't. You might miss valuable information about the patient's chief complaint—the reason for the call. If all else fails, give the patient an opportunity to write responses to your questions.

Obesity. Regardless of the cause of your patient's obesity, your primary responsibility is to provide thorough and professional medical care. Conduct an extensive medical history, keeping in mind the chronic medical conditions commonly associated with obesity.

Obese patients often mistakenly blame signs and symptoms of an untreated illness on their weight. Obtain a complete history of the symptoms and the activities the person was doing when they appeared. When doing your patient assessment, you may also have to make accommodations for the person's weight. For example, if the patient's adipose tissue presents an obstruction, you may need to place electrocardiogram (ECG) monitoring electrodes on the arms and thighs instead of on the chest. You may also need to auscultate lung sounds anteriorly on a patient who is too obese to lean forward. In assessing an obese patient, flexibility is the key. Keep in mind that no two patients and no two environments will be just alike.

Positioning an obese patient for transport may prove especially difficult, because many EMS transportation devices are not designed or rated for heavy weights. Always be sure you have enough lifting assistance for the circumstances. Never compromise your health or safety during the transport process. Finally, remember to let the emergency department know that extra lifting assistance and special stretchers will be needed on your arrival.

Paralysis. If your patient depends on a home ventilator, it is important to maintain a patent airway and to keep the ventilator functioning. Also, a paralyzed patient may have been breathing through a tracheostomy for some time. Therefore, you should keep suction nearby in case the person experiences an airway obstruction. You may also need to use a bag-valve-mask unit to transport the patient to the ambulance if the ventilator does not transport easily. If the patient has suffered a recent spinal cord injury, halo traction may still be intact. Be sure to stabilize the traction before transport.

While performing your physical assessment, you may come across a colostomy appliance. This device is necessary when the patient does not have normal bowel function from paralysis of the muscles needed for proper elimination. Be sure to take any other assisting devices, such as canes or wheelchairs, so the patient can get around once out of your care. For more on acute interventions for people with physical disabilities and other chronic care patients, see Chapter 8 in this volume.

Developmental Disabilities. Unless a patient has Down syndrome or lives in a group home or other special residential setting, it may be difficult to recognize someone with a developmental disability. The disability may become obvious only when you start your interview, and even then the person may be able to provide adequate information. Remember that persons with developmental disabilities can recognize body language, tone, and disrespect just like anyone else. Treat them as you would any other patient, listening to their answers, particularly if you suspect physical or emotional abuse. As mentioned in previous chapters, people in this group have a higher-than-average chance of being abused, particularly by someone they know.

If a patient has a severe cognitive disability, you may need to rely on others to obtain the chief complaint and history. In this case, plan to spend a little extra time on the physical assessment, because the patient may not be able to tell you what is wrong. Also, many children or young people with learning disabilities have been taught to be wary of strangers who may seek to touch them. You will have to establish a basis of trust with the patient, perhaps by making it clear that you are a member of the medical community or by asking for the support of a person the patient does trust. Also, some people with developmental disabilities have been judged "stupid" or "bad" for behavior that results in an accident and, therefore, they may try to cover up the events that led up to the call.

©2013 Pearson Education, Inc.
Paramedic Care: Principles & Practice, Vol. 6, 4th Ed.

At all times, keep in mind that a person with a developmental disability may not understand what is happening. The ambulance, special equipment, and even your uniform may confuse or scare him. In cases of severe disabilities, it will be important to keep the primary caregiver with you at all times, even in the back of the ambulance. Talk to patients with disabilities in terms they will understand and demonstrate what you are doing, as much as possible, on yourself or your partner.

Arthritis. Treatment for arthritis includes aspirin, nonsteroidal anti-inflammatory drugs (NSAIDS), and/or corticosteroids. You should be able to recognize the side effects of these medications because you may be called on to treat a medication side effect rather than the disease. NSAIDS can cause stomach upset and vomiting, with or without bloody emesis. Corticosteroids, such as prednisone, can cause hyperglycemia, bloody emesis, and decreased immunity. You should also take note of all the patient's medications so you do not administer a medication that can interact with the ones already taken by the patient.

When transporting arthritis patients, keep in mind their high level of discomfort. Use pillows to elevate affected extremities. The most comfortable patient position might not be the best position to start an IV, but try to make the patient as comfortable as possible. Special padding techniques may be required because of the patient's arthritis.

Cancer. Management of the patient with cancer can present a special challenge to the paramedic. Many patients undergoing chemotherapy treatments become neutropenic. This is a condition in which chemotherapy creates a dangerously low level of neutrophils, the white blood cells responsible for the destruction of bacteria and other infectious organisms. Frequently during chemotherapy the neutrophils are destroyed along with the cancer cells, severely increasing the patient's risk for infection.

If patients have recently undergone chemotherapy, assume that they are neutropenic. Reduce their exposure to infection as much as possible. Remember that, once infected, a neutropenic patient can quickly go into septic shock, sometimes in a matter of hours. For this reason, keep a mask on such patients during both transport and transfer at the emergency department.

Also keep in mind that cancer patients' veins may have become scarred and difficult to access as a result of frequent IV starts, blood draws, and caustic chemotherapy transfusions. A patient with cancer may also have an implanted infusion port, found just below the skin, with the catheter inserted into the subclavian vein or brachial artery. This port is accessed for infusion of chemotherapy drugs or IV fluids using sterile technique. You need special training to use these implanted ports and should not attempt to access them unless you have such training. Local protocols usually dictate whether an EMS provider may access one of these devices.

Patients may request that you do not start a peripheral IV if their port can be accessed at the hospital. In such cases, you need to consider if your IV is a lifesaving necessity that cannot wait or if the patient can indeed wait for access at the emergency department.

Patients with cancer may also have a peripheral access device, such as a Groshong catheter or Hickman catheter, which have has access ports that extend outside the skin. In this situation, it may simply be a matter of flushing the line and then hooking up your IV fluids to this external catheter. Whatever you decide to do, involve the patient in the decision-making process whenever possible. Patients with cancer lose much control over their lives during treatment, so it is important for them to maintain as much control over their EMS care as possible.

Cerebral Palsy. In treating patients with cerebral palsy, keep this fact in mind: Many people with athetoid and diplegic cerebral palsy are highly intelligent. Do not automatically assume that a person with cerebral palsy cannot communicate with you. Also, as you might expect, many cerebral palsy patients rely on special devices to help them with their mobility. Diplegic patients, for example, may be dependent on wheelchairs.

When transporting patients with cerebral palsy, make accommodations to prevent further injury. If they experience severe contractions, patients may not rest comfortably on a stretcher. Use pillows and extra blankets to pad extremities that are not in normal alignment. Have suction available if a patient drools. If a patient has difficulty communicating, make sure that the caregiver helps in your assessment. Be alert for patients with cerebral palsy who sign. If you do not know sign language, try to find someone who does and alert the emergency department.

Cystic fibrosis. Obtaining a complete medical history is important to the recognition of a patient with cystic fibrosis. In treating these patients, remember that they have been chronically ill for their entire lives. The last thing they may want is another trip to the hospital. For this reason, transport can be difficult for both the patient and family members. To allay their fears, keep in mind the developmental stage of your patient. A child with CF is still a child, so recall everything you have learned about the treatment and comforting of pediatric patients.

Because of the high probability of respiratory distress in a patient with CF, some form of oxygen therapy may be necessary. You may need to have a family member or caregiver hold blow-by oxygen, rather than using a mask, if that is all the patient will tolerate. Suctioning may be necessary to help the patient clear the thick secretions from the airway. CF patients may be taking antibiotics to prevent infection and using inhalers or Mucomyst to thin their secretions. Make sure that you take along all medications so that the hospital staff can continue with the patient's regimen.

Multiple sclerosis. The initial signs of MS are usually temporary. However, they return and become more frequent and long lasting. As the symptoms progress, they become more permanent, leading to a weak extremity or paralysis. Over time, some patients may become bedridden and lose control of bladder function. Eventually an MS patient may develop a lung or urinary infection, which may lead to death. As with other chronically ill patients, people with MS may experience mood swings and seek medical attention for their feelings.

Transport of a patient with MS to the hospital may require supportive care, such as oxygen therapy. Make sure the patient is comfortable, by helping to position the person as necessary. Do not expect patients with MS to walk to the ambulance. Even if they normally are ambulatory, they may be in a more weakened state than usual. Again, be sure to bring assistive devices, such as a wheelchair or cane, so the patient can maintain as much independence as possible.

Muscular dystrophy. Because MD is a hereditary disease, you should obtain a complete family history. You should also note the particular muscle groups that the patient cannot move. Again, because patients with MD are primarily children, choose age-appropriate language. Respiratory support, such as oxygen, may be needed, especially in the later stages of the disease.

Poliomyelitis. Many patients with polio or post-polio syndrome try to maintain their independence. They may insist on walking to the ambulance but should not be encouraged to do so. The idea of hospitalization will frustrate them, because many polio survivors have memories of spending months or even years in hospitals as children. Unlike other patients with chronic illnesses, most people who have had polio do not require frequent trips to the hospital. Therefore, this may be their first time in the back of an ambulance. Try to alleviate their anxiety as much as possible.

Previous head injuries. Obtaining a medical history from these patients is very important, especially if you are responding to a traumatic event. Note any new symptoms the patient may be having or the recurrence of old ones. Conduct the physical assessment slowly. If the patient cannot speak, look for obvious physical signs of trauma or for facial expressions of pain. Transport considerations will depend on the condition for which you were called. However, information about the previous head injury, if you can obtain it, should be an important part of the patient's transfer.

Spina bifida. Symptoms depend on which part of the spinal cord is protruding through the back. The patient may have paralysis of both lower extremities and lack of bowel or bladder control. A large percentage of children born with spina bifida have hydrocephalus, which is the accumulation of fluid in the brain. If the patient has hydrocephalus, a shunt will need to be inserted to help drain off the excess fluid. Permanent disabilities cannot be assessed until the defect is surgically corrected.

When treating patients with spina bifida, keep several things in mind. Recent research has shown that between 18 and 73 percent of children and adolescents with spina bifida have latex allergies. For safety, assume that all patients with spina bifida have this problem. In transporting a patient with spina bifida, be sure to take along any devices that aid the patient. If you are called to treat an infant, safe transport to the hospital should be done in a car seat unless contraindicated.

Myasthenia gravis. A patient with myasthenia gravis may complain of a complete lack of energy, especially in the evening. The disease commonly involves muscles in the face. You may note eyelid drooping or difficulty in chewing or swallowing. The patient may also complain of double vision.

©2013 Pearson Education, Inc.
Paramedic Care: Principles & Practice, Vol. 6, 4th Ed.

In severe cases of myasthenia gravis, a patient may experience paralysis of the respiratory muscles, leading to respiratory arrest. These patients will, of course, need assisted ventilations en route to the emergency facility. For patients with less severe cases, accommodations will vary based on presentation.

4. Adapt your approach to communication, history taking, assessment, and management to interact effectively with patients from a variety of cultural backgrounds. p. 207

With American society becoming more diverse, instead of less diverse, the ability to tolerate cultural differences will become an important part of your professionalism as a paramedic.

From time to time, you may encounter a patient who will make a decision about medical care with which you do not agree. For example, Christian Scientists do not believe in human intervention in sickness through the use of drugs or other therapies. You cannot force these patients to accept an IV or to take nitroglycerin if they are having chest pains. Remember, the patient who has decision-making capabilities has a right to self-determination. You should, however, obtain a signed document indicating informed refusal of consent.

Accommodation of a culturally diverse population will require patience and, in some cases, ingenuity. If your patient does not speak English, and you do not speak the patient's language, communication may be a problem. You may need to rely on a family member to act as an interpreter or on a translator device, such as a telephone language line for non-English-speaking people. In such cases, be sure to notify the receiving facility of the need for an interpreter.

5. Anticipate the special needs and concerns of patients with financial challenges. p. 208

One of the exciting parts of a career in EMS is the opportunity to meet people of all backgrounds. You have the chance to get out into the street and see how people live, work, and play. This allows you to help and educate people who may not otherwise have access to health care. Become familiar with public hospitals and clinics that provide services to people without money or adequate insurance coverage. Calm a patient's fears by discussing this and providing as much helpful information as you can. In providing care, always keep this guideline in mind: Treat the patient, not the financial condition the patient is in.

6. Document relevant observations and information regarding patients with special challenges. pp. 196–208

Your documentation regarding patients with special challenges should possess the same basic attributes as any other documentation. Appropriate terminology, proper spelling, accepted abbreviations and acronyms, and accurate times are essential. A description of the patient's history, environment, assessment, and interventions are equally important. All personnel, including interpreters and home care providers, and resources involved in the call must be documented. The record must be accurate and precise, free of jargon, and neatly written. Corrections should be made properly, including the use of an addendum when appropriate.

Case Study Review

Reread the case study on page 196 in Paramedic Care: Special Patients; *then, read the following discussion.*

This case study draws attention to the effect of preexisting physical impairments—paralysis and weakness from polio and post-polio syndrome—on a call involving a fall. Although the medics were called to treat the patient for the fall, the physical impairments affected their assessment and management of the patient.

Preexisting impairments can complicate assessment. Mrs. Wade, for example, had lived with the effects of polio and post-polio syndrome for so long that she initially forgot to mention her paralyzed right leg and the weakness in her left arm. Fortunately, the patient was alert and could provide plenty of assistance. For example, she indicated that the pain in her hip and shoulder were new and in all likelihood fall related. When questioned about her leg, Mrs. Wade also could identify the cause, plus add further information on post-polio syndrome. However, not all calls involving challenged patients may be this clear cut, especially in cases where the patient is not alert and/or is unable to communicate clearly. For this reason, it is important to be aware of the way in which common mental and physical impairments present themselves.

As with many challenged patients, Mrs. Wade had done some planning. She had hidden an extra key outside the house and carried a mobile phone with her. Some patients may also wear Lifeline® transmitter devices around their necks. These devices, which operate with the press of a button, are usually linked with either an answering service or a hospital, which in turn notifies an EMS dispatch agency to respond. Again, not all cases will be so well scripted. The patient may be locked inside a house or apartment, and you will have to gain access. Or a great deal of time may pass before the patient or somebody else summons help.

The impairments cited by Mrs. Wade—polio and post-polio syndrome—are not as commonly encountered as other impairments mentioned in this chapter. Never feel embarrassed about not knowing about every medical condition. Ask the patient for information. You will be surprised how much information the patient or caregiver can provide.

Finally, treatment was not confined to fall-related injuries. The weakness caused by post-polio syndrome was addressed by placing the patient's left arm in a sling. It relieved some of the pain related to the post-polio syndrome and made the patient more comfortable. During packaging and transport, it might have been helpful to use pillows and blankets to pad the scoop or stretcher to increase patient comfort even more.

Content Self-Evaluation

MULTIPLE CHOICE

_____ 1. The two main types of deafness are
   A. tinnitus and Meniere's disease.
   B. conductive and sensorineural.
   C. partial and sudden.
   D. clinical and nonclinical.
   E. temporary and complete.

_____ 2. A middle ear infection frequently associated with upper respiratory infection is
   A. labyrinthitis.
   B. otitis media.
   C. presbycusis.
   D. otomycosis.
   E. cerumen.

_____ 3. During the patient interview and physical exam, hearing deficits may be mistaken for
   A. head injury.
   B. intoxication.
   C. transducer infection.
   D. effusion syndrome.
   E. drug overdose.

_____ 4. When communicating with a deaf patient, consider all of the following strategies, EXCEPT
   A. speaking slowly in a normal voice.
   B. using a high-pitched voice to speak directly into the patient's ear.
   C. reducing background noise.
   D. using a pen and paper.
   E. putting a stethoscope on the patient and speaking into it.

_____ 5. The term for removal of the eyeball after trauma, such as a penetrating injury, or certain kinds of illnesses is
   A. retinal detachment.
   B. enucleation.
   C. optic chiasm.
   D. orbitotomy.
   E. corneal abrasion.

_____ 6. Diabetes can slowly lead to a loss of a vision as a result of
   A. degeneration of the optic nerve.
   B. disorders in the blood vessels leading to the retina.
   C. degeneration of the eyeball.
   D. cytomegalovirus (CMV).
   E. retinitis.

©2013 Pearson Education, Inc.
Paramedic Care: Principles & Practice, Vol. 6, 4th Ed.

_____ 7. When approaching a patient with a seeing-eye dog in a harness, pet the dog to show that you mean no harm to its owner.
- **A.** True
- **B.** False

_____ 8. All of the following are types of speech impairments, EXCEPT
- **A.** congenital disorders.
- **B.** language disorders.
- **C.** fluency disorders.
- **D.** articulation disorders.
- **E.** voice production disorders.

_____ 9. A language disorder that can be caused by a stroke or brain injury is known as
- **A.** amnesia.
- **B.** ataxia.
- **C.** aphagia.
- **D.** aphasia.
- **E.** aphonia.

_____ 10. Stuttering is an example of a(n)
- **A.** dyslexic disorder.
- **B.** fluency disorder.
- **C.** auditory disorder.
- **D.** vocal cord disorder.
- **E.** voice production disorder.

_____ 11. If the adipose tissue on an obese patient presents an obstruction, you may need to place ECG monitoring electrodes on the
- **A.** chest and back.
- **B.** hands and feet.
- **C.** arms and back.
- **D.** neck and chest.
- **E.** arms and thighs.

_____ 12. A quadriplegic patient has been paralyzed from the waist down.
- **A.** True
- **B.** False

_____ 13. Depression and psychoses are examples of
- **A.** mental and emotional impairments.
- **B.** developmental disabilities.
- **C.** visual impairments.
- **D.** articulation disorders.
- **E.** pathological challenges.

_____ 14. People with Down syndrome are at risk of developing
- **A.** cataracts.
- **B.** blindness.
- **C.** early Alzheimer's disease.
- **D.** heart defects.
- **E.** all of the above.

_____ 15. Fetal alcohol syndrome (FAS) is sometimes confused with Down syndrome because they both
- **A.** produce similar facial characteristics.
- **B.** are caused by alcohol consumption during pregnancy.
- **C.** are preventable birth defects.
- **D.** cause death at an early age.
- **E.** produce hyperactivity.

_____ 16. A preventable disorder caused by alcohol consumption during pregnancy is
- **A.** JRA.
- **B.** FAS.
- **C.** ACE.
- **D.** TIA.
- **E.** PE.

_____ 17. It is not uncommon for children with juvenile rheumatoid arthritis (JRA) to suffer complications involving the spleen or liver.
- **A.** True
- **B.** False

_____ 18. Cancer patients receiving chemotherapy are at high risk for
- **A.** syncope.
- **B.** infection.
- **C.** altered mental status.
- **D.** weight gain.
- **E.** diminished sense of pain.

_____ 19. If a cancer patient has an implanted infusion port, you can generally hook up your IV fluids to this port.
   A. True
   B. False

_____ 20. When caring for cerebral palsy patients, you may need to
   A. treat them as if they have a spinal injury.
   B. change the order of the initial assessment.
   C. use pillows and blankets to pad unaligned extremities.
   D. anticipate brief periods of apnea.
   E. both A and D.

_____ 21. Most of the cystic fibrosis patients that you see will be
   A. adults in their 30s and 40s.
   B. elderly patients over age 60.
   C. infants 1 year old and younger.
   D. children and adolescents.
   E. women between the ages of 20 and 40.

_____ 22. A group of hereditary disorders characterized by progressive weakness and wasting of muscle tissue is known as
   A. poliomyelitis.   D. cystic fibrosis.
   B. spina bifida.   E. muscular dystrophy.
   C. multiple sclerosis.

_____ 23. A congenital abnormality in which a large percentage of children are born with hydrocephalus is
   A. Down syndrome.   D. fetal alcohol syndrome.
   B. cerebral palsy.   E. cystic fibrosis.
   C. spina bifida.

_____ 24. A person with spina bifida would be less likely to have
   A. accumulation of fluid on the brain. D. loss of bowel control.
   B. loss of bladder control.   E. paralysis on one side of the body.
   C. paralysis of the lower extremities.

_____ 25. Research has shown that between 18 and 73 percent of children and adolescents with _____ have latex allergies.
   A. cerebral palsy   D. spina bifida.
   B. myasthenia gravis   E. Down syndrome
   C. poliomyelitis

_____ 26. Common complaints from a patient with myasthenia gravis include
   A. chronic fatigue or lack of energy.
   B. nausea and headache.
   C. shortness of breath and heart palpitations.
   D. dizziness and loss of appetite.
   E. unsteady gait and double vision.

_____ 27. When a patient refuses treatment because of religious reasons, you should
   A. call the police to intervene.
   B. administer treatment and document your reasons.
   C. ask the person to reconsider his religious views.
   D. obtain a signed refusal of treatment and transportation form.
   E. leave the scene.

_____ 28. Accommodation of a culturally diverse population requires
   A. patience.   D. use of translators.
   B. ingenuity.   E. all of the above.
   C. respect.

©2013 Pearson Education, Inc.
Paramedic Care: Principles & Practice, Vol. 6, 4th Ed.

_____ **29.** When treating people with communicable diseases, you should take additional precautions beyond those required by departmental policy.
   A. True
   B. False

_____ **30.** If a homeless person is unable to afford medical bills, it is your job to help the patient get health care regardless of his financial situation.
   A. True
   B. False

MATCHING

Write the letter of the term in the space provided next to the appropriate description.

A. labrynthitis   **I.** neutropenic

B. conductive deafness   **J.** enucleation

C. motor aphasia   **K.** cerumen

D. deafness   **L.** colostomy

E. diabetic retinopathy **M.** mucoviscidosis

F. sensorineural deafness **N.** presbycusis

G. sensory aphasia   **O.** glaucoma

H. otitis media

_____ **31.** An inability to hear

_____ **32.** Progressive hearing loss that occurs with aging

_____ **33.** Middle ear infection

_____ **34.** Group of eye disorders that result in increased intraocular pressure on the optic nerve

_____ **35.** Earwax

_____ **36.** Occurs when the patient cannot speak but can understand what is said

_____ **37.** A surgical diversion of the large intestine through an opening in the skin where the fecal matter is collected

_____ **38.** A condition that results in an abnormally low white blood cell count

_____ **39.** Caused when there is a blocking of the transmission of the sound waves through the external ear canal to the middle or inner ear

_____ **40.** Slow loss of vision as a result of damage done by diabetes

_____ **41.** Occurs when a patient cannot understand the spoken word

_____ **42.** Inner ear infection that causes vertigo, nausea, and an unsteady gait

_____ **43.** Removal of the eyeball after trauma or illness

_____ **44.** Caused by the inability of nerve impulses to reach the auditory center of the brain because of nerve damage either to the inner ear or to the brain

_____ **45.** Cystic fibrosis of the pancreas resulting in abnormally viscous mucoid secretion from the pancreas

Special Project

Continuing Education: Using the Internet

The Internet is a very useful source of information about many of the conditions and diseases discussed in this chapter. Take a moment to browse the Internet and locate the websites for each of the following advocacy organizations. Record each URL, or website address, in the space provided. Don't stop with this list. Expand your references, adding the Internet addresses for other organizations, including local chapters in your area.

AGENCY	WEBSITE
American Cancer Society	
American Foundation for the Blind	
American Obesity Association	
American Speech-Language-Hearing Association	
Arthritis Foundation	
Cystic Fibrosis Foundation	
Down Syndrome Society	
Multiple Sclerosis Association of America	
Muscular Dystrophy Association	
Myasthenia Gravis Foundation of America	
National Health Care for the Homeless Council	
National Organization on Fetal Alcohol Syndrome	
Polio Experience Network	
Spina Bifida Association of America	
United Cerebral Palsy	

©2013 Pearson Education, Inc.
Paramedic Care: Principles & Practice, Vol. 6, 4th Ed.

Acute Interventions for the Chronic Care Patient

Review of Chapter Objectives

In each chapter of the workbook, we identify the objectives and the important elements of the text content. You should review these items and refer to the pages listed if any points are not clear.

After reading this chapter, you should be able to:

1. Define key terms introduced in this chapter.   p. 212

Knowing and being able to apply the key terms in each chapter is critical to understanding chapter concepts. Write the list of key terms. Then write the definition of each one in your own words. Check your understanding by confirming the definitions in the text glossary. Correct any misunderstandings. Create a study aid by writing each key term on the front of an index card and the definition on the back. Use the cards to quiz yourself, or to have someone quiz you.

2. Describe factors that have contributed to the increase in home health care.   pp. 213–214

Numerous factors have promoted the growth of home care in recent years, including enactment of Medicare in 1965, the advent of health maintenance organizations, improved medical technology, and studies showing improved recovery rates and lower costs with home care. Supporters of home health care point out that patients often recover faster in the familiar environment of their homes than in the hospital. They also emphasize differences in the cost of home care versus hospital care. The savings promised by home health care continue to speed the dismissal of patients from hospitals and nursing homes.

3. Relate the epidemiology of patients receiving home health care to paramedics' knowledge needs with respect to home health care.   pp. 214–215

As patients and their families assume greater responsibility for their own treatment and recovery, the likelihood of advanced life-support (ALS) intervention for the chronic care patient increases. Calls may come from the patient, the patient's family, or a home health care provider.

In home care settings, you can expect to encounter a sometimes dizzying array of devices, machines, medications, and equipment designed to provide anything from supportive to life-sustaining care. As a paramedic, you should become familiar with the basic functions of the common home care devices and, just as important, recognize the underlying need for them. The failure or malfunction of this type of equipment has the potential to become a life-threatening or life-altering event. New technologies and machines are being developed constantly. It is your responsibility to stay informed of these changes and the assessment complications that may be involved with the use of each device.

4. **Anticipate the psychosocial concerns of patients receiving home health care and of their family members.** pp. 220–221

Patients require home care for a variety of reasons. Some simply do not need to recover from an injury or illness in a hospital or a rehabilitation facility. Their home care is transitory and their condition usually improves. Other patients have chronic conditions that require varying degrees of home assistance so the patients can live relatively normal lives. These patients usually adjust to their illnesses or disabilities, but never completely recover. Still other patients have terminal illnesses that may or may not involve complicated supportive measures. Their conditions are expected to worsen, and these patients may in fact be waiting to die.

All these situations require sensitivity to the special needs of the patient and consideration of the people involved in the patient's care. Strong emotions may emerge during the call. A previously manageable condition may have suddenly become unmanageable or more complicated. Unlike in a hospital, the patient or home care provider cannot push a button and summon immediate help. Instead, they often summon you, the ALS provider.

5. **Describe common reasons why paramedics are summoned to assist patients receiving home health care.** pp. 215–217

A number of situations may involve you in the treatment of a home care patient: equipment failure, unexpected complications, absence of a caregiver, need for transport, inability of the patient or caregiver to operate a device, and more. As already mentioned, you might also be called on to provide emotional support or intervention. Taking responsibility for an illness or an ill family member can be a stressful and overwhelming experience. Some people may be ill equipped to deal with complicated directions, mechanical problems, or the stress of long-term care. Do not minimize their frustrations or allow these frustrations to interfere with your care. Your primary role as an ALS provider is to identify and treat any life-threatening problems.

6. **Anticipate common complications that occur with various types of home health care equipment.** p. 217

Home care equipment has the normal limitations of any machine. The power may go out and stop the machine from functioning. The machine may break and/or need maintenance. Some machines, if inoperative, can create a life threat to a patient. Common examples include home ventilators, oxygen delivery systems, apnea monitors, and home dialysis machines.

In cases of equipment malfunction, you may be called on to take the place of a device (such as a ventilator) or to treat problems that have arisen as a result of the malfunction. Even the malfunction of a glucometer for a diabetic can be a difficult situation for some patients to handle, especially if they suspect hypoglycemia. Your job is to assess the problem and take the appropriate actions.

7. **Recognize home health care patients with signs and symptoms of infection and sepsis.** p. 233

You should always maintain a high index of suspicion for infection in a home care patient with a decreased immune response, either from poor general health or a specific disease. Be particularly alert to infections in patients with indwelling devices such as gastrostomy tubes, peripherally inserted central catheter (PICC) lines, Foley catheters, or colostomies. Also remember that patients with limited lung function or tracheotomies cannot clear their airways easily, putting them at a higher risk of lung infections.

Patients who have decreased sensorium from a variety of conditions may have wounds and ulcers that they are unaware of, especially if they have been bedridden or inactive for long periods of time. Surgically implanted drains or wound closures may become infected without the patient realizing it. A bed-bound patient may also develop decubitus wounds, pressure sores, or bedsores. If these problems are not identified or treated, they can progress from a generalized infection to gangrene and sepsis.

In identifying infections, look for the following general signs: redness and/or swelling, especially at the insertion site of an indwelling device; purulent discharge at the insertion site; warm skin at the insertion site; and fever.

Infection at the cellular level is called cellulitis and is not life threatening. When an infection spreads systemically, however, it can lead to sepsis—a serious medical emergency. This may cause a patient's immune system to fail, resulting in septic shock. Signs and symptoms of sepsis include redness at an insertion site, fever, altered mental status, poor skin color or turgor, signs of shock, vomiting, and diarrhea.

Keep in mind that home care patients may already be receiving treatment for a generalized infection that has in fact worsened or spread. Inquire whether a pattern of deterioration has been seen by the caregiver or home care provider. In cases of septic shock, ALS treatment is mainly supportive. Provide fluid for hypotension and necessary airway and oxygen support.

8. Describe the need to interact with other health care professionals when responding to patients receiving home health care. pp. 217–218

An important source of information is the home care provider, whether that person is a nurse, nurse's aide, family member, or friend. Remember that this person usually knows the patient better than anyone else. The provider will often spot subtle changes in the patient's condition that may seem insignificant to the outsider. In assessing the patient, it is crucial that you listen carefully to what this person says.

Home care providers are often health care professionals, but be sensitive in questioning their training or background. You must obtain certain information to care for your patient, and the home care provider may be the only source you have for critical items such as the patient's baseline mental status. If you meet resistance, either from the home care provider's lack of training or from a misunderstanding of your needs, try rephrasing your question or using less technical language. At all times, keep in mind the presence of the patient. Involve him in the questioning process.

9. Adapt techniques of scene size-up, patient assessment, and patient care interventions to the special situations of patients receiving home health care. pp. 219–221

Assessment of the home care patient follows the same basic steps as any other patient: scene size-up, primary assessment, secondary assessment, reassessment, and continued management. However, you will need to modify your mind-set for the home care patient—that is, observe for conditions that you might not ordinarily look for in the general population.

As with any call, your assessment of the scene begins before you get out of your vehicle. In the case of home care patients, note any special equipment you may observe upon entering the home. This will alert you to any possible chronic problems that the patient might have. Special hazards that you may face in a home care situation include infectious wastes, medical supplies such as needles, and potentially dangerous equipment. Another important part of the scene size-up involves an evaluation of the patient's environment. Also note the condition of the patient's specific medical devices. Remember that you not only have a responsibility to treat the patient, but to act as an advocate. Remain alert to signs of abuse and/or neglect.

As you approach the patient, begin your primary assessment by observing the patient's general appearance, skin color and quality, quality of respiration, and level of distress. Also note any medical equipment that the patient may be currently using. As you continue to assess the patient for the ABCs, try to ascertain from the primary care provider (if present) a baseline presentation for the patient. Were you called because an existing condition has gotten worse? Or are you here for a new problem? As with any patient, treat the problem as you see it! Once you have established the patient's baseline, assess for changes from the norm. Airway and breathing are always your first concern, followed by circulation. If there are any serious threats to the ABCs, you must treat them. If you are unable to stabilize the patient, complete your rapid assessment and transport immediately. In noncritical patients, you might take the opportunity to compare vital signs with the bedside records, if they are kept. The focus of your exam should be on the chief complaint and how it might relate to the patient's chronic condition.

If your patient has a preexisting altered mental status, such as dementia or Alzheimer's disease, you must have a good understanding of his normal mentation before transport. Remember that home care patients, especially older or terminal patients, are fearful of being removed from the home environment. This can trigger depression, which in turn worsens a preexisting altered mental status.

In preparing your history, take into account any long-term medical problems (i.e., the conditions that necessitated home care) and the specific events that led to the current crisis. Use the home health history and written orders from the physician, if available. The patient or family may have a discharge sheet with valuable information. As mentioned, talk to the health care provider and to the patient.

Keep in mind that eating habits, fluid intake, and minor illnesses or injuries can have a dramatic effect on a seriously ill homebound patient. Have a high index of suspicion for any new conditions that the patient may be developing.

10. **Consider the existence of a DNR/DNAR or other physician orders or instructions when caring for patients receiving home health care.** p. 221

In the case of home care patients, you may more commonly encounter do not resuscitate (DNR) orders, do not attempt resuscitation (DNAR) orders, living wills, and so on. Ascertain whether these documents are in place before beginning any lifesaving treatments. If that information is unavailable, act in the best interests of the patient. Also, keep in mind that a DNR or DNAR doesn't mean that you have to withhold all treatment. However, you must read the specific instructions contained within the advance directives and consult with medical control. Advance directives are designed to prevent unwanted treatment and invasion to the body when natural death or dying occurs. However, many people who have advance directives can be treated in crisis situations and recover. You must use your judgment on a case-by-case basis to determine what qualifies as a resuscitative or life-sustaining measure.

Local protocols may also vary with respect to DNRs, DNARs, living wills, and durable power of attorney documents. Be sure that you are familiar with these legal statements and their implications for care of the terminally ill.

11. **Address the special assessment and equipment troubleshooting needs for patients with each of the following situations:**

a. **Respiratory problems** pp. 222–229

As you approach the patient, look at the effort required to breathe. Observe for head bobbing, retractions, respiratory rate, tripod posturing, pursed lips, quality and effort of speech, cyanosis, and depth of respiration. Listen for sounds of wheezing or crackles. Note any devices or medications that the patient is currently using. Immediately assess the patient's mental status by talking to him as you approach. Patients will indicate understanding with their eyes even if they are unable to speak as a result of dyspnea. Note the number of words the patient can speak without stopping for a breath. Rapidly confirm the patient's baseline respiratory effort and mental status from the home care worker, if present.

Next, auscultate the lungs to identify the type of problem that the patient may be having and to determine tidal volume. Look at the patient's chest to spot any irregularities, retractions, or abdominal breathing. You can use pulse oximetry as an adjunct to your assessment, but do not rely on it alone. If the patient has poor peripheral circulation, pulse oximetry may not give an accurate reading.

Finally, complete your assessment by considering the full range of problems that might have caused the patient's current complaint. Whenever assessing a home care patient, you must remain vigilant for complications other than the chronic medical condition being treated at home.

Tracheostomy. The most common problems faced by tracheostomy patients include blockage of the airway by mucus and a dislodged cannula. The patient can usually clear the obstructing mucus by coughing. Sometimes suctioning, either by the patient or by the caregiver, will suffice. Cannulas can become dislodged by patient movement, or, in the case of children, by their growth. In assessing a child with a cannula problem, find out when it was last changed. Children can also have their stoma blocked by foreign objects that enter by accident or are put there by a sibling. Other complications include infection of the stoma, drying of the tracheal mucus leading to crusting or bleeding, and tracheal erosion from an overinflated cuff (causing necrosis).

©2013 Pearson Education, Inc.
Paramedic Care: Principles & Practice, Vol. 6, 4th Ed.

If the tracheostomy patient is on a ventilator, you must rapidly determine if the problem is with the ventilator or with the airway itself. If the problem is simply a loose fitting or disconnected tube, fix it. If the problem is not immediately apparent, do not waste time trying to troubleshoot the machine; remove the tubing, connect the bag-valve device to the trach connector, and ventilate.

If the problem is with the patient's airway, you will need to clear it. If the patient is hypoxic, always hyperventilate before suctioning. Be sure to evaluate any postural or positional considerations. If the patient is slumped over, straighten him up. Remember to ensure that ventilations are directed downward into the lungs, not upward into the mouth.

If you are unable to ventilate, clearing the airway is your first priority. Visualize as much of the airway as possible and check for obstructions. If none are visible, introduce a suction catheter and suction while withdrawing—no more than 10 to 15 seconds for an adult, 5 seconds for a child. Again, always hyperventilate before and after suctioning.

If it appears that the inner cannula is blocked or dislodged, you may remove it. If cuffed, you must first deflate the cuff. Connect a 10-mL syringe to the cuff valve and withdraw the air. If a syringe is unavailable, you can cut off the valve and the air will escape. You can then remove the inner cannula, hyperventilate, and continue to suction as needed.

If necessary, you may intubate the stoma. The inner cannula must always be removed first. Use an appropriately sized tube to pass through the outer cannula, and advance so the endotracheal (ET) cuff (if a cuffed tube is used) is 1 to 2 cm inside the trachea. Inflate the cuff and verify placement by auscultating the epigastrium and both lungs. Add an end-tidal CO_2 device to the end of the tube. Pulse oximetry should also be used to monitor patient oxygenation.

Ventilatory devices. Positive end-expiratory pressure (PEEP), continuous positive airway pressure (CPAP), and bilevel positive airway pressure (BiPAP) are three ventilator options that add pressure at various times in the respiratory cycle. They may be used by full-time or part-time ventilator patients. Keep in mind that the danger of pneumothorax exists because of the increased pulmonary pressure. Take this into account during your assessment of PEEP.

Ventilatory problems are traditionally easy to fix in the prehospital environment. If a home ventilator fails, you should begin manual PPV immediately. The failure may be easy to remedy, such as in the case of unplugged power cords or a temporary loss of electricity. If you are trained to work with the ventilator, you can adjust the settings to restore or improve ventilations. However, if you are unfamiliar with the ventilator, play it safe and support ventilations with your own equipment.

Oxygen. As with ventilation, oxygenation problems are also generally easy for EMS providers to fix. First, assess the patency of the patient's home oxygen delivery system. The power may be off, the tubing damaged, or the oxygen supply depleted. You can adjust the flow rate of an intact home oxygen delivery system or replace it with your own system.

b. **Vascular access devices**   pp. 229–230

Vascular access devices (VADs) are used to provide any parenteral treatment on a long-term basis. Patients may have chemotherapy, hemodialysis, peritoneal dialysis, total parenteral nutrition (TPN) feedings, or antibiotic therapy provided through a VAD.

The most common complications result from various types of obstructions. A thrombus may form at the catheter site, or an embolus may lodge there after formation elsewhere in the body. Inactivity increases the risk for clot formation. Other obstructive problems include catheter kinking and catheter tip embolus.

With central venous access devices, you should always be aware of the potential for an air embolus. The devices provide a clear pathway for air to enter central circulation. Signs and symptoms of an air embolus include headache, shortness of breath with clear lungs, hypoxia, chest pain, other indications of myocardial ischemia, and altered mental status

Of course, any device implanted in the body has a risk of infection or hemorrhage. Look for redness, swelling, tenderness, localized heat, or discharge at a potentially infected catheter site. Because these catheters provide a channel into the central circulation, patients may quickly become septic, especially if they are weakened or immunosuppressed.

c. **Cardiovascular problems**   p. 230

Many chronic care patients receive treatment for a wide variety of cardiac conditions. You may be called to intervene in the following situations: post–myocardial infarction recovery, postcardiac surgery, heart transplant, congestive heart failure (CHF), hypertension, implanted pacemaker, atherosclerosis, and congenital malformation (pediatric).

Home care for the cardiac patient can consist of oxygen, monitoring devices, and regular visits by a home health care provider. You can expect to find a variety of medications associated with the specific cardiac problem: bedside cardiac monitors (for adults and children), diagnostic devices such as a halter monitor, and possibly a defibrillator.

d. Gastrointestinal and genitourinary problems and devices   pp. 230–233

Most complications related to urinary tract support devices result from infection or device malfunctions. Infection is a very common problem with urinary tract devices because the area is rich with pathogens and because the catheter provides a pathway directly into the body. Remain alert to foul-smelling urine or altered urine color, such as tea-colored, cloudy, or blood-tinged urine. Also look for signs and symptoms of systemic infection, or urosepsis, because urinary infections can quickly spread in the immunocompromised patient. Suprapubic catheters or urostomies may also have infections at the abdominal wall site. You should note redness, swelling, heat, discharge, or loss of skin integrity.

Device malfunctions typically include accidental displacement of the device, obstruction, balloon ruptures in devices that use a balloon as an anchor, or leaking collection devices. Changes in the patient's anatomy, such as a shortened urinary tract or tissue necrosis, can also cause malfunctions. Ensure that the collection device is empty and record the amount of urine output. Look for kinks or other obstructions in the device, and make sure that the collection bag is placed below the patient.

Complications from gastrointestinal (GI) tract devices include tube misplacement, obstruction, and infection. Because misplaced tubes can obstruct the airway or GI system, you should always ensure device patency if you have doubts about placement of the tube. First, have the patient speak to you. If he cannot speak, the tube may be in the airway and need to be removed. Second, to ensure patency of an NG tube, use a 60-mL syringe to insert air into the stomach. Use your stethoscope to listen over the epigastrum for air movement within the stomach. A low-pitched rumbling should be heard. You may also note stomach contents spontaneously moving up the tube or they may be aspirated with a 60-mL syringe. In such cases, patients may be repositioned to return patency, or the device may be reinserted.

Tubes are also prone to obstructions. Colostomies may become clogged or otherwise obstructed. Feeding tubes can become clogged because of the thick consistency of supplemental feedings or pill fragments. As a result, the tubes may require irrigation with water. In addition, the thick consistency of food may cause bowel obstructions or constipation.

As might be expected, ostomies can become infected (or lose skin integrity from pressure). Look for signs and symptoms of skin or systemic infection. In addition, remember that digestive enzymes may leak from various ostomies and begin to digest the skin and abdominal contents.

e. Maternal and newborn care   pp. 233–234

For the mother, postpartum bleeding and embolus (especially after a caesarean section) are the most common complications. Management of an embolus would be the same as with any patient with a similar complaint. Postpartum bleeding can be a serious condition. Management steps include massage of uterus, if not already contracted; administration of fluids to correct hypotension; administration of certain medications, such as Pitocin (if ordered); and rapid transport to the hospital, if necessary.

Mothers may also experience postpartum depression. In such cases, women may have difficulty caring for both themselves and their newborns. In extreme cases, babies have been neglected or even harmed.

When entering the home, be sensitive to the needs of the parents. First-time mothers and/or fathers may be inexperienced in child rearing and may call EMS for what a more experienced parent might regard as normal. It is important that you always take any parent's concerns seriously, and if no medical support is needed, provide emotional reassurance.

Infants with recognized problems may already be receiving home care. They may have cardiac or respiratory abnormalities or other congenital defects. Premature or low-birth-weight babies, as well as babies with any number of respiratory disorders, are at risk for sleep apnea. Such babies may wear apnea monitors around their chests so that an alarm sounds at any pause in their breathing pattern. Some infants may also be on pulse oximetry. If you are summoned because of an alarm and find a normal breathing pattern, still encourage the parents or caregivers to have the baby examined as soon as possible.

©2013 Pearson Education, Inc.
Paramedic Care: Principles & Practice, Vol. 6, 4th Ed.

Newborns may also be discharged from the hospital with an undetected cardiac or respiratory condition. Signs and symptoms of cardiac or respiratory insufficiency include: cyanosis, bradycardia (<100 beats per minute), crackles, and respiratory distress. In such cases, resuscitation should be initiated immediately. Management should be toward respiratory support with a BVM or intubation, as necessary. If any newborn has a heart rate < 80 beats per minute despite 30 seconds or more of oxygenation, start cardiopulmonary resuscitation (CPR). Preserve warmth and obtain a record from the parents of feeding intake since birth. If the infant has not been feeding or has been vomiting with diarrhea, the infant may be dehydrated. In this case, a fluid bolus of 20 mL/kg is indicated. If a peripheral IV cannot be obtained in two attempts or 2 minutes, obtain access via the intraosseous route. If blood sugar is below 80 mg/dL administer $D_{10}W$ at a dosage of 0.5 mg/kg.

For a newborn with infection or septicemia, look for fever, tachycardia, and irritability. If septicemia progresses to septic shock, you should initiate resuscitation as previously described.

Children who have serious, long-term health problems are usually cared for by their parents at home, with or without the help of a home care professional. Commonly found medical therapies for children who are home care patients include mechanical ventilators, IV medications or nutrition, oxygen therapy, tracheostomies, feeding tubes, pulse oximeters, and apnea monitors.

When dealing with children, remember to keep the parents or caregivers informed of your assessment and treatment plans. Children quickly pick up on a person's emotions. As a result, it is part of your job to act in a supportive and controlled manner. Calming a child could make a huge difference in the long-term effects of the current episode.

f. Hospice care
pp. 234–235

The goal of hospices is to provide palliative or comfort care, rather than curative care. This is a very different role from that of most other branches of the health care profession, including EMS. For an ALS team, care is usually geared toward aggressive and lifesaving treatment. A hospice team, on the other hand, seeks to relieve symptoms, manage pain, and give patients control over the end of their lives. It is important to remember that these patients have, for the most part, exhausted or declined curative resources.

Involvement in a hospice situation can be a difficult and stressful call. In most cases, family members, caregivers, and health care workers have been instructed to call a hospice rather than EMS. However, you may be summoned for intervention, particularly in situations involving transport. You should always keep in mind that the hospice patient is in the end stages of his disease and has already expressed wishes to withhold resuscitation. However, even a valid DNR order should not prevent you from performing palliative and/or comfort care.

In a hospice, you need to establish communication with the home health care worker as quickly as possible. Your inclination may be to intubate, start a line, or administer medications. However, as noted, palliative care supersedes curative care. A hospice worker, when faced with the end stage of a disease, may do nothing, in accordance with the patient's wishes. Therefore, it is vital that you gain a clear understanding of these wishes, whether through a family member or a written document. If you are called to the house, it is your responsibility to respect the wishes of the patient and the ideals of hospice care. In a hospice situation, family members might panic at a patient's imminent death and appropriate care might involve support for the family rather than resuscitation of the patient.

Case Study Review

Reread the case study on pages 212–213 in Paramedic Care: Special Patients; *then, read the following discussion.*

The case study draws attention to the assessment and management of a chronic condition commonly found in a prehospital setting—chronic obstructive pulmonary disease (COPD), an illness that is subject to acute exacerbation during the end stage.

Patient assessment in the case begins as soon as the paramedics arrive on the scene. A quick survey of the room reveals the presence of several oxygen bottles on the floor and a patient on a nasal cannula. The EMS team immediately knows that their patient has already been treated on a home care basis for some kind of respiratory disorder, which conforms to the description supplied by the dispatcher ("elderly male, short of breath").

Signs and symptoms clearly point to severe respiratory distress: use of the accessory muscles for breathing, anxiety, dyspnea, prolonged expiration with pursed lips, and the inability to speak in full sentences. Auscultation of lung sounds (diminished breathing in all fields with inspiratory and expiratory wheezes), vital signs, and patient history confirm this suspicion.

Mr. Casey—who is in end-stage COPD—has a valid prehospital DNR, which he shows the paramedic. This document affects the actions taken by the prehospital care providers. As indicated in the case study, the DNR precludes intubation, so they continue with pharmacological interventions only. Because local protocols vary on advanced directives, it is important for you to become familiar with these well ahead of facing a real-life situation such as the one in this case.

Content Self-Evaluation

MULTIPLE CHOICE

_____ 1. All of the following factors have promoted the growth of home care in recent years, EXCEPT
    A. enactment of Medicare.
    B. the advent of managed care.
    C. an increase in malpractice lawsuits.
    D. improved recovery rates.
    E. improved medical technology.

_____ 2. As patients assume greater responsibility for their own treatment and recovery, the likelihood of ALS intervention for the chronic care patient increases.
    A. True
    B. False

_____ 3. Common reasons for ALS intervention in the treatment of a home care patient include all of the following, EXCEPT
    A. inability to operate a device.   **D.** need for transport.
    B. absence of a caregiver.   **E.** pain management.
    C. equipment failure.

_____ 4. Home care providers can be of great assistance to EMS crews because they
    A. have more experience in the field of prehospital medicine.
    B. will often spot subtle changes in the patient's condition.
    C. will easily grasp technical medical language.
    D. have legal authority to speak for the patient.
    E. both C and D.

_____ 5. A home care patient is likely to decompensate and will go into crisis more quickly than the general population.
    A. True
    B. False

_____ 6. Common causes of cardiac decompensation—a true medical emergency leading to shock—include all of the following, EXCEPT
    A. acute myocardial infarction.   **D.** sepsis.
    B. stroke.   **E.** heart transplant.
    C. cardiac hypertrophy.

_____ 7. One reason that diabetics get gangrene is due to slowed circulation to the extremities.
    A. True
    B. False

_____ 8. Home interventions such as peritoneal dialysis can alter electrolytes.
    A. True
    B. False

©2013 Pearson Education, Inc.
Paramedic Care: Principles & Practice, Vol. 6, 4th Ed.

9. Signs and symptoms of sepsis in a patient with an indwelling device can include
   A. cyanosis at the infection site.
   B. fever.
   C. increased urination.
   D. cool skin at the insertion site.
   E. all of the above.

10. The ability of the skin to return to normal appearance after being subjected to pressure is called
    A. capillary refill.
    B. tenting.
    C. turgor.
    D. diaphoresis.
    E. hypertrophy.

11. Conditions that may be treated in a home care setting include
    A. brain or spinal trauma.
    B. arthritis.
    C. AIDS.
    D. transplants.
    E. all of the above.

12. Examples of commonly used medical devices in the home care setting include all of the following, EXCEPT
    A. glucometers.
    B. tracheostomies.
    C. apnea monitors.
    D. heart/lung machines.
    E. indwelling IV sites.

13. The matrix for injury prevention developed by William Haddon include all of the following steps, EXCEPT
    A. prevent the creation of the hazard to begin with.
    B. reduce the amount of the hazard brought into existence.
    C. increase the release of an already existing hazard.
    D. modify the basic qualities of the hazard.
    E. separate the hazard and that which is to be protected by a barrier.

14. It is a serious mistake to arrive on the scene with a "takeover" mentality that all but eliminates the home care provider.
    A. True
    B. False

15. In responding to any home care situation, you should remember that
    A. any bed-bound patient may have pressure sores.
    B. hospital beds, wheelchairs, or walkers may be contaminated by body fluid.
    C. medical wastes may not be properly contained.
    D. sharps may be present.
    E. all of the above.

16. In assessing home care patients, the focus of your physical exam should be on the patient's chronic condition.
    A. True
    B. False

17. Of the following acute home care situations, the one LEAST commonly encountered by paramedics is
    A. respiratory disorders.
    B. end stages of a hospice patient.
    C. cardiac problems.
    D. GI/GU disorders.
    E. use of vascular access devices.

18. When providing intervention to home care patients with chronic respiratory diseases, remember that they usually have a low-dosing regimen, which may make them more responsive to their medications.
    A. True
    B. False

19. In treating home care patients with cystic fibrosis (CF), most patients will probably be
  A. over age 65.
  B. between 40 and 60 years old.
  C. of almost any age.
  D. under age 40.
  E. infants.

20. Which of the following is an advantage of oxygen therapy for the home care patient?
  A. It is relatively easy to manage.
  B. Most patients tolerate it easily.
  C. Oxygen therapy adds to the quality of life.
  D. Oxygen prevents hypoxic states.
  E. All of the above.

21. If a buzzer goes off on an oxygen concentrator, you would mostly likely suspect
  A. faulty tubing.
  B. a leak in the tank.
  C. a dirty or plugged humidifier.
  D. power failure.
  E. either A or C.

22. Routine care of a tracheostomy includes all of the following, EXCEPT
  A. keeping the stoma clean and dry.
  B. removing the device daily.
  C. frequent suctioning.
  D. changing the ventilator hose routinely.
  E. periodically changing/cleaning the inner cannula.

23. Which of the following ventilatory options are you LEAST likely to find in a home care setting?
  A. PEEP
  B. CPAP
  C. BiPAP
  D. poncho-wrap
  E. both A and C

24. Patients with VADs will be much more prone to bleeding disorders than the general population.
  A. True
  B. False

25. The most common complication found in patients with VADs results from
  A. an embolus.
  B. dehydration.
  C. a thrombus.
  D. hypertension.
  E. both A and C.

26. The most commonly used device for urinary tract dysfunction is a(n)
  A. Texas catheter.
  B. urostomy.
  C. Foley catheter.
  D. suprapubic catheter.
  E. condom catheter.

27. The most common complications related to urinary tract support devices result from
  A. obstructions.
  B. device malfunctions.
  C. infections.
  D. misplacement of devices.
  E. both B and C.

28. If you have any doubts about the placement of a nasogastric feeding tube, your first step should be to
  A. listen for air movement within the stomach.
  B. use a 60-mL syringe to insert air into the stomach.
  C. have the patient speak to you.
  D. irrigate the tube with water.
  E. immediately remove the tube.

29. In terms of providing care, the goal of hospices closely resembles the goal of EMS services.
  A. True
  B. False

©2013 Pearson Education, Inc.
Paramedic Care: Principles & Practice, Vol. 6, 4th Ed.

_____ **30.** The stages in the grief process for both the patient and those left behind are
  A. depression, bargaining, guilt, anger, and acceptance.
  B. anger, denial, bargaining, guilt, and acceptance.
  C. denial, bargaining, anger, acceptance, and guilt.
  D. bargaining, denial, anger, guilt, and acceptance.
  E. denial, anger, depression, bargaining, and acceptance.

MATCHING

Write the letter of the term in the space provided next to the appropriate description.

A. hypertrophy   **F.** cellulitis

B. hemoptysis   **G.** gangrene

C. exocrine   **H.** turgor

D. demylenation   **I.** cor pulmonale

E. emesis   **J.** sensorium

_____ **31.** Destruction or removal of the myelin sheath of nerve tissue; found in Guillain-Barré syndrome

_____ **32.** Death of tissue or bone, usually from an insufficient blood supply

_____ **33.** Disorder involving external secretions

_____ **34.** An increase in the size of an organ or structure caused by growth rather than by tumor

_____ **35.** Ability of the skin to return to normal appearance after being subjected to pressure

_____ **36.** Sensory apparatus of the body as a whole; also that portion of the brain that functions as a center of sensations

_____ **37.** Inflammation of cellular or connective tissue

_____ **38.** Expectoration of blood arising from the oral cavity, larynx, trachea, bronchi, or lungs

_____ **39.** Vomitus

_____ **40.** Congestive heart failure secondary to pulmonary hypertension

SHORT ANSWER

Write out the terms that each of the following abbreviations/acronyms stands for in the space provided.

41. PEEP _____

42. CPAP _____

43. BIPAP _____

44. COPD _____

45. ARDS _____

46. PPV _____

47. VAD _____

48. PICC _____

49. DNAR _____

50. CHF _____

Special Project

Find out the names and telephone numbers of home care agencies and hospices in your area. Inquire about the resources/services that they provide and record the information in the following spaces.

HOME CARE AGENCIES		
Name of agency	Contact number	Services provided

HOSPICE AGENCIES		
Name of agency	Contact number	Services provided

Now take one more step. Make a copy of this information and carry it aboard the ambulance or write the phone numbers in the pocket reference that you carry in your uniform pocket!

©2013 Pearson Education, Inc.
Paramedic Care: Principles & Practice, Vol. 6, 4th Ed.

SPECIAL PATIENTS
Content Review
Content Self-Evaluation

Chapter 1: Gynecology

_____ 1. Which of the following structures is part of the external female genitalia?
   A. Ovary
   B. Perineum
   C. Uterus
   D. Vagina
   E. Fallopian tube

_____ 2. An elastic canal that connects the internal and external female genitalia is the
   A. ureter.
   B. urethra.
   C. vagina.
   D. vulva.
   E. fallopian tube.

_____ 3. The distance from the symphysis pubis to the fundus can be used to calculate
   A. duration of premenstrual cycle.
   B. gestational length in weeks.
   C. length of menses.
   D. time since menopause.
   E. age of the patient.

_____ 4. The layer of the uterine wall where the fertilized egg implants is the
   A. dermametrium.
   B. cyclometrium.
   C. myometrium.
   D. perimetrium.
   E. endometrium.

_____ 5. Which of the following hormones is released by the ovaries?
   A. Estrogen
   B. Follicle-stimulating hormone
   C. Gonadotropin
   D. Luteinizing hormone
   E. Thymosin

_____ 6. The menstrual cycle generally lasts
   A. 2 weeks.
   B. 28 days.
   C. 7 days.
   D. 9 months.
   E. 3 weeks.

_____ 7. The onset of ovulation that establishes female sexual maturity is known as
   A. menarche.
   B. menopause.
   C. menses.
   D. menstruation.
   E. menace.

_____ 8. The onset of ovulation usually begins between the ages of
   A. 8 and 12.
   B. 10 and 14.
   C. 12 and 16.
   D. 14 and 18.
   E. 16 and 20.

_____ 9. The _____ phase of the menstrual cycle terminates with ovulation.
   A. ischemic
   B. menstrual
   C. proliferative
   D. secretory
   E. fallow

____ 10. Which process occurs during the proliferative phase of the menstrual cycle?
   A. Drop in estrogen level
   B. Rupture of small endometrial blood vessels
   C. Shedding of the endometrium
   D. Thickening of the endometrium
   E. Endometrium becomes pale

____ 11. The condition in which a woman has severe depression symptoms, irritability, and tension before menstruation is called
   A. premenstrual syndrome.   D. dyspareunia.
   B. dysmenorrhea.   E. menarche.
   C. premenstrual dysphoric disorder.

____ 12. The term used to describe the number of times a woman has been pregnant is
   A. gravida.   D. parity.
   B. gravity.   E. completa.
   C. paridy.

____ 13. The easiest means by which an EMS provider can estimate menstrual flow is
   A. cervical palpation.
   B. the testimony of the patient.
   C. direct observation.
   D. the saturation of one tampon or pad.
   E. the number of tampons or pads used.

____ 14. Which of the following questions is LEAST likely to get an accurate response from a female who is complaining of abdominal pain?
   A. Are you currently menstruating?
   B. Are you sexually active?
   C. Could you be pregnant?
   D. Have you ever experienced this pain before during menses?
   E. Have you experienced dizziness?

____ 15. At 5 months (approximately 20 weeks) of gestation, the uterus is palpable
   A. midway between the umbilicus and the symphysis pubis.
   B. above the symphysis pubis.
   C. just below the xiphoid process.
   D. at the level of the umbilicus.
   E. midway between the umbilicus and the xiphoid process.

____ 16. The most common cause of nontraumatic abdominal pain is
   A. cystitis.   D. ruptured ovarian cyst.
   B. mittelschmerz.   E. endometriosis.
   C. pelvic inflammatory disease.

____ 17. A female patient reports frequent urination and dysuria. This is probably due to
   A. cholecystitis.   D. dyspareunia.
   B. cystitis.   E. endometritis.
   C. dysmenorrhea.

____ 18. Severe abdominal pain associated with ovulation is
   A. cystitis.   D. cholecystitis.
   B. endometriosis.   E. mittelschmerz.
   C. endometritis.

____ 19. Which condition often mimics signs and symptoms of severe pelvic inflammatory disease (PID)?
   A. Endometriosis   D. Ruptured ovarian cyst
   B. Endometritis   E. Cholecystitis
   C. Mittelschmerz

©2013 Pearson Education, Inc.
Paramedic Care: Principles & Practice, Vol. 6, 4th Ed.

_____ **20.** A condition in which endometrial tissue is found outside the uterus is
    A. ectopic pregnancy.   **D.** eschar.
    B. endometriosis.   **E.** mittelschmerz.
    C. endometritis.

_____ **21.** Signs and symptoms of uterine fibroids include all of the following EXCEPT
    A. vaginal bleeding between periods.   **D.** swelling.
    B. light periods.   **E.** pain during intercourse.
    C. abdominal fullness.

_____ **22.** A female reports that during aggressive intercourse she felt a sudden and sharp tearing sensation. She is now bleeding from the external genitalia, although the bleeding is minimal. Management should include all of the following EXCEPT
    A. asking the woman to hold a dressing over the area and apply direct pressure.
    B. establishing an IV and beginning fluid resuscitation, if indicated.
    C. expediting transport to the emergency department.
    D. packing the vagina with sterile dressings.
    E. applying a chemical cold pack over the hematoma.

_____ **23.** Flunitrazepam is the classic "date rape" drug, but any medication that alters mental status, including alcohol, can be used.
    A. True.
    B. False.

_____ **24.** The most important management for a victim of a sexual assault is
    A. aggressive questioning and management.
    B. discouraging the patient from dressing, as this may taint evidence.
    C. examining the genitalia.
    D. providing psychological and emotional support.
    E. promptly summoning law enforcement officials.

_____ **25.** When completing your documentation on a sexual assault victim
    A. state the patient's remarks accurately.
    B. document any evidence turned over to the hospital staff and the name of the individual to whom you gave it.
    C. do not include your opinions as to whether rape occurred.
    D. objectively state your observations of the patient's physical condition, environment, or torn clothing.
    E. all of the above.

Chapter 2: Obstetrics

_____ **26.** Fertilization of the ovum usually occurs in the
    A. cervix.   **D.** uterus.
    B. fallopian tubes.   **E.** perineum.
    C. ovaries.

_____ **27.** A change in the reproductive system during pregnancy is that
    A. mammary glands decrease in number.
    B. secretion of estrogen causes sloughing of the endometrial lining.
    C. the uterus contains about 16 percent of the total maternal blood volume.
    D. uterine connective tissue stiffens to allow for support of the fetus.
    E. dissolution of a mucous plug occurs in the cervix.

_____ **28.** The normal duration of pregnancy is _____ from the first day of the mother's last menstrual period.
    A. 36 weeks   **D.** 44 weeks
    B. 40 weeks   **E.** 48 weeks
    C. 42 weeks

____ **29.** Fetal heart tones can be detected by the _____ week of gestation.
  A. 8th
  B. 12th
  C. 16th
  D. 20th
  E. 28th

____ **30.** By which week of gestation is a baby considered term?
  A. 20th
  B. 25th
  C. 32nd
  D. 38th
  E. 40th

____ **31.** Which structure allows for mixing of blood between the right and left atria?
  A. Ductus arteriosus
  B. Ductus venosus
  C. Foramen ovale
  D. Umbilical vein
  E. Umbilical artery

____ **32.** The ductus arteriosus connects which two structures?
  A. Inferior vena cava and aorta
  B. Pulmonary artery and aorta
  C. Pulmonary vein and aorta
  D. Superior vena cava and aorta
  E. Superior vena cava and pulmonary artery

____ **33.** All of the following are typical causes of vaginal bleeding during pregnancy EXCEPT
  A. abortion.
  B. abruptio placentae.
  C. ectopic pregnancy.
  D. placenta previa.
  E. prolapsed umbilical cord.

____ **34.** A naturally occurring expulsion of the fetus prior to viability, generally due to chromosomal abnormalities, that may occur before the 12th week of gestation is a(n)
  A. inevitable abortion.
  B. missed abortion.
  C. spontaneous abortion.
  D. threatened abortion.
  E. term abortion.

____ **35.** Which sign or symptom differentiates eclampsia from preeclampsia?
  A. Chronic hypertension
  B. Gestational diabetes
  C. Seizure
  D. Supine hypotensive disorder
  E. None of the above

____ **36.** One way to minimize supine hypotension in the pregnant patient is to
  A. allow her to sit in the semi-Fowler's position.
  B. place her in a full Trendelenburg position.
  C. position her tilted slightly to the right.
  D. sit her upright with feet dangling.
  E. place her in the left lateral recumbent position.

____ **37.** All of the following may cause preterm labor EXCEPT
  A. exercise.
  B. infection.
  C. multiple gestation.
  D. placenta previa.
  E. diabetes.

____ **38.** Which of the following medications is considered a tocolytic for preterm labor?
  A. Magnesium sulfate
  B. Oxytocin
  C. Pitocin
  D. Racemic epinephrine
  E. Dextran

____ **39.** Crowning of the fetus occurs during the _____ stage.
  A. dilatation
  B. expulsion
  C. placental
  D. puerperium
  E. postpartal

©2013 Pearson Education, Inc.
Paramedic Care: Principles & Practice, Vol. 6, 4th Ed.

_____ 40. Although it was once a common practice, suctioning of the nasopharynx in neonates without obvious obstruction is no longer recommended.
   A. True.
   B. False.

_____ 41. Immediate care of the newborn should include all of the following EXCEPT
   A. assessing the neonate using APGAR scoring.
   B. drying the infant.
   C. immediately ventilating the infant with 100 percent oxygen.
   D. repeated suctioning of the mouth and nose with respiratory diffulty and thick meconium.
   E. covering the infant with a dry receiving blanket.

_____ 42. Which of the following is considered a normal delivery?
   A. Breech presentation   D. Vertex position
   B. Occiput posterior   E. Limb presentation
   C. Prolapsed cord

_____ 43. Management of breech presentation delivery includes all of the following EXCEPT
   A. gently pulling on the infant's legs to facilitate delivery of the head.
   B. inserting a gloved hand into the vagina to allow for unrestricted respirations.
   C. placing the mother in supine position with legs flexed.
   D. supporting the infant's trunk.
   E. rotating the infant's body so that the shoulders are in anterior-posterior position.

_____ 44. The proper position for the expectant mother in the event of a limb presentation is
   A. flat prone.   D. supine with legs flexed.
   B. prone in a knee-to-chest fashion.   E. the Trendelenburg position.
   C. supine with legs flat and forced together.

_____ 45. The most common cause of postpartum hemorrhage is
   A. uterine atony.   D. uterine rupture.
   B. uterine hypertrophy.   E. uterine abscess.
   C. uterine inversion.

Chapter 3: Neonatology

_____ 46. Complication(s) that may result from hypoxia during the birth process include
   A. persistent fetal circulation.   D. hypovolemia.
   B. spinal cord defects.   E. both A and C.
   C. hypothermia.

_____ 47. Persistent fetal circulation is best described as which of the following?
   A. Cardiovascular flow causing pink extremities and blue trunk
   B. Postdelivery bradycardia
   C. Bypass of the respiratory system
   D. Ongoing asphyxia, also called secondary hypoxia
   E. Umbilical circulation continuing after delivery

_____ 48. The congenital condition where the tongue is large, the jaw is small, and the patient has a cleft palate is
   A. Pierre Robin syndrome.   D. enhanced cleft palate.
   B. choanal atresia.   E. none of the above.
   C. meningomyelocele.

_____ 49. Heat loss from the newborn occurs through which of the following routes?
   A. Evaporation   D. Radiation
   B. Convection   E. All of the above
   C. Conduction

____ **50.** The third tier of the pediatric resuscitation pyramid includes which of the following?

    A. Drying   **D.** Oxygen

    B. Warming   **E.** Tactile stimulation

    C. Suctioning

____ **51.** A newborn infant presents with peripheral cyanosis and signs of respiratory distress. Your exam reveals a small, flat abdomen with bowel sounds present in the chest. Heart sounds are displaced to the right. You suspect

    A. ductus arteriosus.   **D.** an omphalocele.

    B. Pierre Robin syndrome.   **E.** a congenital defect.

    C. a diaphragmatic hernia.

____ **52.** Seizures in neonatal patients are often the result of

    A. developmental abnormalities.   **D.** metabolic disturbances.

    B. drug withdrawal.   **E.** all of the above.

    C. fever.

____ **53.** All of the following are findings in a hypothermic newborn EXCEPT

    A. tachycardia.

    B. acrocyanosis, respiratory distress or apnea.

    C. initial irritability, lethargy in later stages.

    D. skin cool to the touch, particularly in the extremities.

    E. inability to shiver.

____ **54.** Vomiting in the neonate is most frequently an isolated incident, unrelated to other pathology.

    A. True

    B. False

____ **55.** The most common cause of cardiac arrest in a newborn is

    A. congenital abnormalities.   **D.** hypoxia.

    B. meconium aspiration.   **E.** diaphragmatic hernia.

    C. hypovolemia.

Chapter 4: Pediatrics

____ **56.** Care of the pediatric patient includes care for the child's parents or caregivers.

    A. True

    B. False

____ **57.** The child's most common response to illness or injury is fear. Common fears of children include all of the following, EXCEPT fear of

    A. separation.   **D.** being hurt.

    B. disfigurement.   **E.** automobiles.

    C. the unknown.

____ **58.** It is a good idea to let a parent remain with the small child during care and transport.

    A. True

    B. False

____ **59.** What percentage of birth weight is lost by the newborn in the first few days of life?

    A. None   **D.** 20 percent

    B. 5 percent   **E.** 35 percent

    C. 10 percent

____ **60.** All of the following conditions place a pediatric patient at risk of cardiopulmonary arrest EXCEPT

    A. heart rate of 160 in a 7-year-old child.   **D.** fever with petechiae.

    B. respiratory rate greater than 60.   **E.** altered level of consciousness.

    C. heart rate above 180 in a 5-year-old child.

©2013 Pearson Education, Inc.
Paramedic Care: Principles & Practice, Vol. 6, 4th Ed.

_____ **61.** Wh,at size cuff would you use when taking a pediatric blood pressure?
   A. Use a cuff with its width equal to the width of the arm.
   B. Use a cuff with its width equal to two-thirds the width of the arm.
   C. Simply assure an adult cuff is tight.
   D. Use an adult cuff but reduce the reading value by 30 percent.
   E. none of the above—pediatric blood pressures are unreliable.

_____ **62.** Mild hypotension is a common and relatively insignificant sign in the pediatric patient.
   A. True
   B. False

_____ **63.** The best size approximation of a nasopharyngeal airway is
   A. use an airway number equal to the patient age in years.
   B. use a #10 French for neonates and a 12 for toddlers.
   C. measure length against the patient's jaw.
   D. size to the external diameter of the child's little finger.
   E. none of the above.

_____ **64.** Nasogastric tube insertion should be considered in the pediatric patient because it relieves gastric distention and improves the adequacy of ventilations.
   A. True
   B. False

_____ **65.** Rapid-sequence intubation is an advanced airway procedure that may be indicated in all of these pediatric patients, EXCEPT a(n)
   A. combative 6-year-old child with head trauma.
   B. 9-year-old child experiencing generalized tonic-clonic seizures.
   C. 8-year-old patient without a gag reflex.
   D. 14-year-old patient attempting suicide by overdose.
   E. vomiting 3-year-old with head trauma from a fall.

_____ **66.** In assessing a pediatric patient for shock, which of the following statements is NOT true?
   A. A smaller absolute volume of loss is needed to cause shock.
   B. A child in shock will always have decreased blood pressure.
   C. Hypotension is an ominous sign of imminent cardiac arrest.
   D. Assessment is based upon clinical signs of tissue perfusion.
   E. A larger relative volume of loss is needed to cause shock.

_____ **67.** The appropriate defibrillation charge for a 15-kilogram pediatric patient is _____ joules per kilogram.
   A. 1 to 2   D. 2 to 5
   B. 1 to 3   E. 3 to 6
   C. 2 to 4

_____ **68.** Being able to recognize the stages of respiratory compromise quickly is paramount for the paramedic. Deteriorating normal mental status, tachypnea, nasal flaring (in infants), and grunting are all signs and symptoms of
   A. respiratory distress.   D. respiratory arrest.
   B. respiratory shunting.   E. all of the above.
   C. respiratory failure.

_____ **69.** Signs of decompensated shock in a pediatric patient include all of the following, EXCEPT
   A. tachycardia.   D. cyanosis.
   B. bradycardia.   E. hypotension.
   C. hypertension.

_____ **70.** If intravenous diazepam cannot be administered to a pediatric patient because intravenous access has not been made, oral diazepam should be administered.
   A. True
   B. False

_____ 71. Which of the following is a likely cause of vomiting in the pediatric patient?
A. Fever
B. Ear infections
C. Gastroenteritis
D. Respiratory infections
E. All of the above

_____ 72. In treating pediatric diabetic patients, remember that most have been taught about their condition and can participate, in varying degrees, in their care.
A. True
B. False

_____ 73. Pediatric patients account for the majority of poisonings treated by EMS.
A. True
B. False

_____ 74. What percentage of pediatric near-drowning survivors exhibit severe neurologic deficits?
A. Less than 5 percent
B. 10 to 20 percent
C. 20 to 25 percent
D. 30 to 35 percent
E. More than 40 percent

_____ 75. Which of the following is NOT true regarding pediatric airway care?
A. The sniffing position best maintains the airway in children over 3 years old.
B. Airway pressures are relatively low.
C. Needle cricothyrotomy is rarely indicated.
D. Gastric tubes are frequently placed to decompress the stomach.
E. It may be necessary to disable the pop-off value on the bag-valve mask (BVM).

_____ 76. Which of the following is NOT a sign of increasing intracranial pressure?
A. Elevated blood pressure
B. Bradycardia
C. Rapid and deep respirations, progressing to slow and deep respirations
D. Constricted pupils
E. Bulging fontanelles

_____ 77. What percentage of pediatric spinal fractures occur at the C1–C2 level?
A. 15 to 20 percent
B. 20 to 25 percent
C. 40 to 50 percent
D. 50 to 60 percent
E. 60 to 70 percent

_____ 78. What percentage of the body's surface does the head and neck receive in the pediatric rule of nines?
A. 9 percent
B. 18 percent
C. 14.5 percent
D. 13.5 percent
E. 6.25 percent

_____ 79. Symptoms of an ALTE include
A. obstruction by a mucus plug.
B. loss of muscle tone.
C. a dislodged tube.
D. infection.
E. all of the above.

_____ 80. Which of the following is LEAST likely to indicate possible child abuse?
A. A fracture in a child under 2 years
B. A greenstick fracture in an 8-year-old
C. Multiple injuries in various stages of healing
D. Intra-abdominal trauma in the young child
E. Injury that does not fit the described mechanism of injury

©2013 Pearson Education, Inc.
Paramedic Care: Principles & Practice, Vol. 6, 4th Ed.

Chapter 5: Geriatrics

____ 81. It is predicted that by 2040, the elderly population will reach 20 percent of the total population.
  A. True
  B. False

____ 82. Which of the following is a federal program that is mostly responsible for paying for medical care for the elderly patient?
  A. Social Security
  B. Medicare
  C. Medicaid
  D. Veteran's Administration
  E. None of the above

____ 83. In the elderly, signs and symptoms are more likely directly related to the disease process causing them.
  A. True
  B. False

____ 84. A contributing factor to decreased medication compliance by the elderly is
  A. polypharmacy.
  B. income limitations.
  C. sensory impairment.
  D. prolonged therapy.
  E. all of the above.

____ 85. Effective continence requires
  A. an anatomically correct GI/GU tract.
  B. a competent sphincter mechanism.
  C. adequate cognition and mobility.
  D. A, B, and C.
  E. A and C only.

____ 86. All of the following are by-products of malnutrition, EXCEPT
  A. vitamin deficiencies.
  B. dehydration.
  C. hypoglycemia.
  D. hyperlipidemia.
  E. both A and B.

____ 87. Factors that complicate the assessment of geriatric patients include
  A. diminished pain perception.
  B. presence of multiple diseases.
  C. failure to report symptoms.
  D. dementia.
  E. all of the above.

____ 88. It is often difficult for the paramedic to differentiate acute from chronic physical findings in the elderly patient.
  A. True
  B. False

____ 89. Common symptoms of senility and organic brain syndrome include all of the following, EXCEPT
  A. delirium.
  B. serenity.
  C. confusion.
  D. restlessness.
  E. hostility.

____ 90. Which of the following statements about the aging process is NOT true?
  A. Chest wall compliance decreases.
  B. The lungs lose their elasticity.
  C. The brain shrinks.
  D. The left ventricular wall thickens.
  E. The skin becomes thicker.

____ 91. Syncope occurring as a result of the body's inability to compensate for movement from the supine position to the seated position or from the seated position to the standing position is known as
  A. cardiac syncope.
  B. vasovagal syncope.
  C. orthostatic syncope.
  D. nocturnal syncope.
  E. vasodepressor syncope.

_____ 92. Risk factors for strokes include all of the following, EXCEPT
   A. atherosclerosis.
   B. hypertension.
   C. atrial fibrillation.
   D. dementia.
   E. immobility.

_____ 93. Allowed to progress, diabetes can result in neuropathy and visual impairment.
   A. True
   B. False

_____ 94. Which of the following is NOT a common cause of seizures in the elderly patient?
   A. Stroke
   B. Mass lesion (tumor or bleed)
   C. Hyperventilation
   D. Alcohol withdrawal
   E. Hypoglycemia

_____ 95. Which of the following is NOT true regarding dementia?
   A. More than 50 percent of nursing home residents have some form of dementia.
   B. Delirium is a form of dementia.
   C. It is a global cognitive impairment.
   D. It is often irreversible.
   E. Alzheimer's disease is a form of dementia.

_____ 96. The primary cause of Parkinson's disease is a neuromuscular disease triggered by a small stroke and related to diet.
   A. True
   B. False

_____ 97. Which of the following is NOT a cause of lower GI bleeding?
   A. Esophageal varices
   B. Diverticulosis
   C. Tumors
   D. Ischemic colitis
   E. Arterio-venous malformations

_____ 98. A significant contributing factor to osteoarthritis in the elderly is
   A. obesity.
   B. inflammatory arthritis.
   C. trauma.
   D. congenital abnormalities.
   E. all of the above.

_____ 99. Which of the following predisposes the elderly to hypothermia?
   A. Previous central nervous system (CNS) disorders such as stroke
   B. Chronic illness
   C. Malnutrition
   D. Drugs that interfere with heat-generation mechanisms
   E. All of the above

_____ 100. Aging results in reduced size and weight of the brain. Which of the following statements about traumatic head injuries in the elderly patient is TRUE?
   A. Signs and symptoms of brain injury appear faster.
   B. Signs and symptoms of brain injury occur more slowly.
   C. Brain injury is less common in elderly patients.
   D. Elderly patients recover more quickly from brain injury.
   E. Brain injuries are less severe in elderly patients.

Chapter 6: Abuse, Neglect, and Assault

_____ 101. A paramedic could potentially identify an abusive family situation by recognizing which of the following generic risk factors?
   A. The children are all in school.
   B. Both parents are employed.
   C. The residence is untidy.
   D. The family is below the poverty level.
   E. All of the children are sick.

_____102. Two signs of domestic elder abuse are
   A. head injury and loss of speech.   D. poor hygiene and loss of appetite.
   B. untreated decubitus ulcers and poor hygiene.   E. good hygiene and bruising.
   C. dementia and loss of freedom.

_____103. Abuse as a child is typically isolated and forgotten once the abused child becomes an adult.
   A. True
   B. False

_____104. Shaken baby syndrome can cause permanent brain damage and may also result in
   A. hair loss.   D. blindness.
   B. malnutrition.   E. cerebral palsy.
   C. chest trauma.

_____105. Hostility, drug abuse, promiscuity, and nightmares are indicative of
   A. mental abuse.   D. neglect.
   B. physical abuse.   E. none of the above.
   C. sexual abuse.

_____106. Liquid Ecstasy, Liquid X, Scoop, and Easy Lay are street names for
   A. Rohypnal.   D. MDMA.
   B. GHB.   E. none of the above.
   C. Ketamine.

_____107. Some of the date rape drugs cause amnesia, thus eliminating or distorting the victim's recall of the assault.
   A. True.
   B. False.

_____108. Paramedics can help the victim of a suspected rape by
   A. assisting the patient with bathing and dressing.
   B. providing a private and safe environment for assessment and care.
   C. treating the patient at the residence without transporting.
   D. avoiding talking about the attack, as it may upset the patient more.
   E. completing a thorough patient assessment, including genitalia.

_____109. The perpetrator of a hate crime targets a particular victim or victims because of the victim's perceived membership in a certain social group.
   A. True
   B. False

_____110. Most hate crimes involve
   A. assault.   D. vandalism.
   B. intimidation.   E. none of the above.
   C. widespread violence.

Chapter 7: The Challenged Patient

_____111. A paramedic can improve communication with a hearing-impaired patient by
   A. addressing the patient face-to-face.
   B. speaking clearly using exaggerated gestures.
   C. making up hand signals the patient recognizes.
   D. talking loudly without using exaggerated gestures.
   E. all of the above.

_____112. Paramedics should always ask permission before touching a service animal, its harness, or its leash.
   A. True
   B. False

____113. A speech disorder characterized by an inability to understand the spoken word is called
- **A.** dysphasia.
- **B.** sensory aphasia.
- **C.** motor aphasia.
- **D.** global aphasia.
- **E.** anuria.

____114. Obesity occurs when a person has an abnormal amount of body fat and a weight _____
_____heavier than is normal for people of the same age, gender, and height.
- **A.** 5 to 10 percent
- **B.** 10 to 20 percent
- **C.** 20 to 30 percent
- **D.** 30 to 40 percent
- **E.** 40 to 50 percent

____115. A traumatic spinal cord injury in the area of C3 to C5 is especially important because it affects the ability to
- **A.** move the legs.
- **B.** move the arms.
- **C.** move the head.
- **D.** breathe.
- **E.** move the fingers.

____116. Fetal alcohol syndrome patients are often born with small eyes with short slits, a small jaw, and a small head.
- **A.** True
- **B.** False

____117. Cancer is a blanket term for many different diseases, each with its own characteristics but having in common the abnormal growth of cells in normal tissue.
- **A.** True
- **B.** False

____118. Which of the following is NOT a common cause of cerebral palsy?
- **A.** Maternal drug overdose
- **B.** Encephalitis
- **C.** Meningitis
- **D.** Head injury
- **E.** Premature birth

____119. Which of the following is true regarding mucoviscidosis?
- **A.** It is also called multiple sclerosis.
- **B.** It is an acquired disorder.
- **C.** It primarily affects the muscular system.
- **D.** It causes a decrease in pancreatic enzymes.
- **E.** All of the above.

____120. Which of the following is a disease of the autoimmune system characterized by chronic weakness in the voluntary muscles?
- **A.** Multiple sclerosis
- **B.** Myasthenia gravis
- **C.** Cystic fibrosis
- **D.** Poliomyelitis
- **E.** Muscular dystrophy

Chapter 8: Acute Interventions for the Chronic Care Patient

____121. According to the National Center for Health Statistics, almost 75 percent of home care patients are members of what age group?
- **A.** Under 18 years old
- **B.** Under 45 years old
- **C.** 45 to 55 years old
- **D.** 55 to 65 years old
- **E.** 65 years or older

____122. Upon arriving at the home of a chronic home care patient, the paramedic should
- **A.** not treat the patient if a home care provider is on the way.
- **B.** assume the home care provider has less training than the paramedic.
- **C.** respectfully get a report from the home care provider on the scene.
- **D.** ask any home care provider to leave the scene.
- **E.** none of the above.

©2013 Pearson Education, Inc.
Paramedic Care: Principles & Practice, Vol. 6, 4th Ed.

_____123. An infection at the cellular level is called cellulitis and is a life-threatening condition requiring acute emergency care.
A. True
B. False

_____124. An acute viral infection that damages the myelin sheath covering peripheral nerves, causing rapid loss of motor function, is
A. multiple sclerosis.
B. cerebral palsy.
C. myasthenia gravis.
D. Guillain-Barré syndrome.
E. cystic fibrosis.

_____125. You are called to the residence of a home care patient with a history of myasthenia gravis. What type of respiratory assistance device might you expect to find?
A. Ventilator
B. Heart/lung machine
C. IV pump
D. Colostomy bag
E. Urinary bag

_____126. The airway ventilator option that adds a small pressure at the end of expiration is
A. CPAP.
B. BiPAP.
C. ADRS.
D. PEEP.
E. all of the above except C.

_____127. The patient with a vascular access device (VAD) such as a PICC line will be on anticoagulant therapy and predisposed to bleeding disorders such as stroke and GI bleeding.
A. True
B. False

_____128. Signs and symptoms associated with VADs and air embolism include all of the following, EXCEPT
A. headache.
B. elevated pulse oximetry readings.
C. chest pain.
D. dyspnea without crackles.
E. altered mental status.

_____129. Care for the postpartum mother with serious hemorrhage should include which of the following?
A. Fundal massage
B. Fluid administration
C. Possible pitocin administration
D. Rapid transport
E. All of the above

_____130. In a newborn discharged from the hospital who is displaying cyanosis, bradycardia (<100 beat per minute), respiratory crackles, and respiratory distress, you should suspect which of the following?
A. Respiratory insufficiency
B. Cardiac insufficiency
C. Hypovolemia
D. Severe infection
E. Both A and B

WORKBOOK ANSWER KEY

Note: Throughout the Answer Key, textbook page references are shown in italics.

Chapter 1: Gynecology

Content Self-Evaluation

MULTIPLE CHOICE

1.	C	*p. 6*	**6.**	B	*p. 8*	**11.**	B	*p. 12*		
2.	B	*p. 6*	**7.**	C	*p. 10*	**12.**	D	*p. 12*		
3.	D	*p. 6*	**8.**	A	*p. 11*	**13.**	C	*p. 11*		
4.	B	*p. 7*	**9.**	E	*p. 11*	**14.**	B	*p. 12*		
5.	D	*p. 7*	**10.**	A	*p. 12*	**15.**	A	*p. 13*		

LABELING THE DIAGRAM

p. 4

A.	Ovary	**D.**	Cervix
B.	Fallopian tube	**E.**	Vagina
C.	Uterus		

SPECIAL PROJECT: Problem Solving: Abdominal Pain

pp. 10–12

1. Focused history elements:
   - SAMPLE and OPQRST
   - Obstetric history: gravida, parity, abortion
   - Gynecological history: past ectopic pregnancies, surgical procedures
   - History of trauma
   - Last menstrual period (LMP)
   - Form of birth control and regularity of use

2. Differential diagnosis possibilities:
   - PID
   - Ruptured ovarian cyst
   - Endometritis
   - Ectopic pregnancy

Chapter 2: Obstetrics

Content Self-Evaluation

MULTIPLE CHOICE

1.	A	*p. 19*	**10.**	A	*p. 27*	**19.**	C	*p. 41*
2.	D	*p. 19*	**11.**	A	*p. 27*	**20.**	A	*p. 38*
3.	E	*p. 22*	**12.**	C	*p. 28*	**21.**	A	*p. 39*
4.	D	*p. 21*	**13.**	B	*p. 30*	**22.**	B	*p. 38*
5.	A	*p. 23*	**14.**	E	*p. 31*	**23.**	B	*p. 39*
6.	C	*p. 24*	**15.**	C	*p. 35*	**24.**	C	*p. 42*
7.	E	*p. 24*	**16.**	B	*p. 34*	**25.**	D	*p. 40*
8.	C	*p. 25*	**17.**	B	*p. 44*			
9.	B	*p. 27*	**18.**	A	*p. 43*			

MATCHING

26.	C	*p. 22*	**30.**	B	*p. 19*	**34.**	I	*p. 33*
27.	E	*p. 19*	**31.**	J	*p. 33*	**35.**	G	*p. 32*
28.	D	*p. 19*	**32.**	F	*p. 32*			
29.	A	*p. 19*	**33.**	H	*p. 24*			

SPECIAL PROJECT: Understanding the Physiological Changes of Pregnancy

pp. 19–22

Reproductive system

Physiological Changes:
- Increased vascularity—one-sixth of total blood volume
- Increased uterine size and capacity—can cause supine hypotensive syndrome and compress vena cava
- Mucus plug blocks cervix to protect fetus
- Mammary glands increase in size and number

EMS Implications:
- Fetal well-being dependent on maternal well-being
- Position mother tilted slightly to the left to minimize hypotension

Respiratory system

Physiological Changes:
- Increased oxygen demand
- Progesterone causes decrease in airway resistance
- Slight increase in respiratory rate
- Rib margins flare to accommodate diaphragmatic elevation due to increased fundal height

EMS Implications:
- Maintain airway
- Administer high-flow, high-concentration oxygen as needed

Cardiovascular system

Physiological Changes:
- Increased cardiac output
- Maternal blood volume increases by 45 percent (slightly more plasma than red blood cells, causing relative anemia)
- Maternal heart rate increases 10 to 15 beats/minute
- Blood pressure initially decreases in first trimester, then rises to near normal during third trimester
- Supine hypotensive syndrome due to weight of gravid uterus compressing the inferior vena cava and impaired venous return

EMS Implications:
- Vital signs should be assessed with patient lying on her left side
- May suffer significant blood loss without significant change in vital signs
- Syncope is relatively common in pregnancy
- Assess amount of reported vaginal bleeding based on number of sanitary pads used (two per hour is significant)
- Anticipate shock based on chief complaint or mechanism of injury
- Overt signs of shock are late and inconsistent

- Initiate vascular access with two large-bore IVs (crystalloid fluids)

Gastrointestinal system

Physiological Changes:

- Nausea and vomiting common in first trimester
- Changed carbohydrate needs
- Peristalsis slows, causing delayed gastric emptying
- Abdominal organs compressed and compartmentalized due to enlarged uterus

EMS Implications:

- MD should evaluate all complaints of abdominal pain
- Assessment is difficult due to compression of organs by uterus, thus "classic signs" of abdominal pathology may be absent or altered
- Potential for regurgitation always present in pregnant patient

Urinary system

Physiological Changes:

- Renal blood flow increases, as does renal tubular absorption
- Glucosuria may result from kidney's inability to reabsorb glucose
- Urinary bladder is displaced anteriorly and superiorly
- Urinary frequency is common due to uterine compression

EMS Implications:

- Glucosuria may indicate the development of gestational diabetes—check blood glucose for any altered mental status during pregnancy
- Displacement of bladder increases risk of traumatic rupture

Musculoskeletal system

Physiological Changes:

- Pelvic joints loosen due to hormonal influence
- Postural changes compensate for anterior uterine growth

EMS Implications:

- Due to loosened joints, pelvis may appear unstable on exam
- Anterior growth may increase incidence of falls due to changed center of gravity

Chapter 3: Neonatology

Content Self-Evaluation

MULTIPLE CHOICE

1.	B	p. 49	4.	E	p. 49	7.	A	p. 51
2.	A	p. 49	5.	B	p. 49	8.	B	p. 53
3.	C	p. 49	6.	A	p. 49	9.	E	p. 53

10.	D	p. 53	19.	A	p. 54	28.	D	p. 60
11.	C	p. 53	20.	E	p. 55	29.	A	p. 60
12.	C	p. 53	21.	A	p. 55	30.	A	p. 62
13.	B	p. 53	22.	B	p. 56	31.	B	p. 63
14.	A	p. 53	23.	B	p. 56	32.	D	p. 63
15.	C	p. 53	24.	D	p. 56	33.	A	p. 65
16.	A	p. 54	25.	B	p. 57	34.	A	p. 66
17.	A	p. 54	26.	A	p. 59	35.	B	p. 66
18.	E	p. 54	27.	B	p. 60			

SPECIAL PROJECT: The APGAR Scale

Part I: TOTAL SCORE = 4

Part II: From top to bottom, items should read—oxygen, bag-mask ventilation, chest compressions, intubation, medications.

Part III: TOTAL SCORE = 9

Chapter 4: Pediatrics

Content Self-Evaluation

MULTIPLE CHOICE

1.	C	p. 72	16.	E	p. 85	31.	C	p. 108
2.	D	p. 72	17.	E	p. 85	32.	E	p. 109
3.	A	p. 72	18.	A	p. 87	33.	C	p. 110
4.	E	p. 73	19.	A	p. 87	34.	A	p. 111
5.	B	p. 73	20.	D	p. 88	35.	D	p. 112
6.	C	p. 74	21.	C	p. 89	36.	B	p. 114
7.	C	p. 74	22.	D	p. 92	37.	A	p. 115
8.	B	p. 75	23.	E	p. 92	38.	B	p. 117
9.	C	p. 79	24.	C	p. 95	39.	C	p. 118
10.	A	p. 79	25.	E	p. 95	40.	C	p. 122
11.	B	p. 79	26.	C	p. 97	41.	C	p. 123
12.	B	p. 79	27.	D	p. 99	42.	C	p. 127
13.	B	p. 80	28.	A	p. 99	43.	E	p. 128
14.	B	p. 81	29.	C	p. 99	44.	D	p. 129
15.	E	p. 83	30.	B	p. 102	45.	C	p. 131

MATCHING

46.	G	p. 130	53.	J	p. 107	60.	I	p. 109
47.	M	p. 130	54.	B	p. 118	61.	E	p. 108
48.	Q	p. 87	55.	F	p. 117	62.	T	p. 79
49.	P	p. 126	56.	O	p. 116	63.	R	p. 72
50.	K	p. 126	57.	N	p. 113	64.	L	p. 74
51.	A	p. 126	58.	H	p. 113	65.	S	p. 114
52.	D	p. 119	59.	C	p. 111			

©2013 Pearson Education, Inc.
Paramedic Care: Principles & Practice, Vol. 6, 4th Ed.

Special Project: Burn Injuries

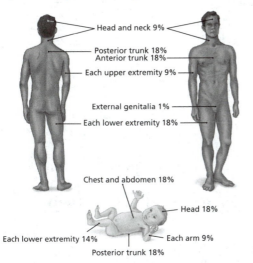

- Head and neck 9%
- Posterior trunk 18%
- Anterior trunk 18%
- Each upper extremity 9%
- External genitalia 1%
- Each lower extremity 18%
- Chest and abdomen 18%
- Head 18%
- Each lower extremity 14%
- Each arm 9%
- Posterior trunk 18%

1. 45 percent
2. 40½ percent
3. Sample Answer: The modified rule of nines for the pediatric patient gives less body surface area to the legs and more to the head of an infant.
4. "rule of palms"

Chapter 5: Geriatrics

Content Self-Evaluation

MULTIPLE CHOICE

1.	B	*p. 140*	4.	C	*p. 141*	7.	D	*p. 142*
2.	C	*p. 140*	5.	D	*p. 142*	8.	C	*p. 142*
3.	E	*p. 141*	6.	B	*p. 142*	9.	E	*p. 144*

10.	A	*p. 144*	34.	B	*p. 151*	58.	B	*p. 160*
11.	C	*p. 146*	35.	A	*p. 152*	59.	A	*p. 161*
12.	A	*p. 147*	36.	D	*p. 152*	60.	B	*p. 162*
13.	B	*p. 146*	37.	A	*p. 152*	61.	D	*p. 162*
14.	C	*p. 146*	38.	C	*p. 152*	62.	C	*p. 163*
15.	D	*p. 146*	39.	A	*p. 153*	63.	D	*p. 164*
16.	E	*p. 146*	40.	C	*p. 154*	64.	A	*p. 165*
17.	A	*p. 147*	41.	C	*p. 155*	65.	B	*p. 166*
18.	B	*p. 147*	42.	B	*p. 155*	66.	B	*p. 167*
19.	B	*p. 147*	43.	B	*p. 155*	67.	A	*p. 166*
20.	C	*p. 147*	44.	E	*p. 155*	68.	B	*p. 167*
21.	D	*p. 147*	45.	A	*p. 156*	69.	E	*p. 167*
22.	A	*p. 148*	46.	E	*p. 146*	70.	B	*p. 168*
23.	E	*p. 148*	47.	A	*p. 157*	71.	A	*p. 169*
24.	A	*p. 149*	48.	B	*p. 156*	72.	A	*p. 170*
25.	C	*p. 149*	49.	B	*p. 158*	73.	C	*p. 171*
26.	E	*p. 149*	50.	A	*p. 158*	74.	B	*p. 172*
27.	C	*p. 149*	51.	E	*p. 158*	75.	D	*p. 173*
28.	E	*p. 149*	52.	A	*p. 159*	76	B	*p. 172*
29.	A	*p. 150*	53.	B	*p. 159*	77.	E	*p. 174*
30.	D	*p. 150*	54.	C	*p. 159*	78.	B	*p. 174*
31.	A	*p. 150*	55.	C	*p. 160*	79.	E	*p. 176*
32.	A	*p. 150*	56.	B	*p. 160*	80.	D	*p. 177*
33.	E	*p. 151*	57.	B	*p. 160*			

MATCHING

81.	J	*p. 164*	86.	O	*p. 175*	91.	K	*p. 164*
82.	G	*p. 170*	87.	I	*p. 163*	92.	N	*p. 179*
83.	A	*p. 162*	88.	B	*p. 162*	93.	D	*p. 162*
84.	H	*p. 161*	89.	C	*p. 162*	94.	F	*p. 163*
85.	M	*p. 166*	90.	L	*p. 163*	95.	E	*p. 148*

SPECIAL PROJECT: Common Age-Related Systemic Changes (*See page 154*)

Body System	Changes with Age	Clinical Importance
Respiratory	Loss of strength and coordination in respiratory muscles Cough and gag reflex reduced	Increased likelihood of respiratory failure
Cardiovascular	Loss of elasticity and hardening of arteries Changes in heart rate, rhythm, efficiency	Hypertension common Greater likelihood of strokes, heart attacks Great likelihood of bleeding from minor trauma
Neurological	Brain tissue shrinks Loss of memory Clinical depression common Altered mental status common Impaired balance	Delay in appearance of symptoms with head injury Difficulty in patient assessment Increased likelihood of falls
Endocrine	Lowered estrogen production (women) Decline in insulin sensitivity Increase in insulin resistance	Increased likelihood of fractures (bone loss) and heart disease Diabetes mellitus common with greater possibility of hyperglycemia
Gastrointestinal	Diminished digestive functions	Constipation common Greater likelihood of malnutrition
Thermoregulatory	Reduced sweating Decreased shivering	Environmental emergencies more common
Integumentary (Skin)	Thins and becomes more fragile	More subject to tears and sores Bruising more common Heals more slowly

continued

Musculoskeletal	Loss of bone strength (osteoporosis)	Greater likelihood of fractures
	Loss of joint flexibility and strength (osteoarthritis)	Slower healing
		Increased likelihood of falls
Renal	Loss of kidney size and function	Increased problems with drug toxicity
Genitourinary	Loss of bladder function	Increased urination/incontinence
		Increased urinary tract infection
Immune	Diminished immune response	More susceptible to infections
		Impaired immune response to vaccines
Hematological	Decrease in blood volume and/or RBCs	Slower recuperation from illness/injury
		Greater risk of trauma-related complications

Chapter 6: Abuse, Neglect, and Assault

Content Self-Evaluation

MULTIPLE CHOICE

1.	B	*p. 183*	8.	C	*p. 186*	15. A	*p. 190*
2.	A	*p. 183*	9.	C	*p. 186*	16. B	*p. 190*
3.	E	*p. 184*	10.	D	*p. 187*	17. A	*p. 192*
4.	C	*p. 184*	11.	E	*p. 187*	18. C	*p. 191*
5.	A	*p. 184*	12.	E	*p. 188*	19. B	*p. 191*
6.	B	*p. 185*	13.	B	*p. 189*	20. A	*p. 191*
7.	B	*p. 185*	14.	B	*p. 189*		

MATCHING

21.	I	*p. 183*	25.	J	*p. 186*	29. A	*p. 183*
22.	E	*p. 192*	26.	D	*p. 186*	30. B	*p. 190*
23.	F	*p. 186*	27.	H	*p. 191*		
24.	C	*p. 190*	28.	G	*p. 183*		

SPECIAL PROJECT: Breaking the Cycle of Abuse: Support Services

The answers will vary with the state, region, or locale where you live. If the information is not readily available in special sections in the telephone book, contact the appropriate agencies, including hospital crisis units, social service agencies, and departments of health.

Chapter 7: The Challenged Patient

Content Self-Evaluation

MULTIPLE CHOICE

1.	B	*p. 197*	11.	E	*p. 200*	21. D	*p. 205*
2.	B	*p. 197*	12.	B	*p. 202*	22. E	*p. 205*
3.	A	*p. 197*	13.	A	*p. 202*	23. C	*p. 207*
4.	B	*p. 198*	14.	E	*p. 203*	24. E	*p. 207*
5.	B	*p. 198*	15.	A	*p. 203*	25. D	*p. 207*
6.	B	*p. 198*	16.	B	*p. 203*	26. A	*p. 207*
7.	B	*p. 199*	17.	A	*p. 203*	27. D	*p. 207*
8.	A	*p. 199*	18.	B	*p. 204*	28. E	*p. 207*
9.	D	*p. 199*	19.	B	*p. 204*	29. B	*p. 207*
10.	B	*p. 200*	20.	C	*p. 205*	30. A	*p. 208*

MATCHING

31.	D	*p. 197*	36.	C	*p. 199*	41. G	*p. 199*
32.	N	*p. 197*	37.	L	*p. 202*	42. A	*p. 197*
33.	H	*p. 197*	38.	I	*p. 204*	43. J	*p. 198*
34.	O	*p. 198*	39.	B	*p. 197*	44. F	*p. 197*
35.	K	*p. 197*	40.	E	*p. 198*	45. M	*p. 205*

SPECIAL PROJECT: Continuing Education: Using the Internet

AGENCY	WEBSITE
American Cancer Society	www.cancer.org
American Foundation for the Blind	www.afb.org
American Obesity Association	www.obesity.org
American Speech-Language-Hearing Association	www.asha.org
Arthritis Foundation	www.arthritis.org
Cystic Fibrosis Foundation	www.cff.org
Down Syndrome Society	www.ndss.org
Multiple Sclerosis Association of America	www.msaa.com
Muscular Dystrophy Association	www.mdausa.org
Myasthenia Gravis Foundation of America	www.myasthenia.org
National Health Care for the Homeless Council	www.nhchc.org
National Organization on Fetal Alcohol Syndrome	www.nofas.org
Polio Experience Network	www.polionet.org
Spina Bifida Association of America	www.sbaa.org
United Cerebral Palsy	www.ucp.org

Chapter 8: Acute Interventions for the Chronic Care Patient

Content Self-Evaluation

MULTIPLE CHOICE

1.	C	*p. 213*	11.	E	*p. 217*	21. D	*p. 225*
2.	A	*p. 213*	12.	D	*p. 217*	22. B	*p. 226*
3.	E	*p. 214*	13.	C	*p. 218*	23. D	*p. 227*
4.	B	*p. 214*	14.	A	*p. 219*	24. A	*p. 230*
5.	A	*p. 215*	15.	E	*p. 219*	25. E	*p. 230*
6.	B	*p. 215*	16.	B	*p. 220*	26. C	*p. 230*
7.	A	*p. 215*	17.	B	*p. 222*	27. E	*p. 231*
8.	A	*p. 215*	18.	B	*p. 222*	28. C	*p. 232*
9.	B	*p. 216*	19.	D	*p. 223*	29. B	*p. 234*
10.	C	*p. 216*	20.	E	*p. 225*	30. E	*p. 235*

©2013 Pearson Education, Inc.
Paramedic Care: Principles & Practice, Vol. 6, 4th Ed.

MATCHING

31.	D *p. 224*	**35.**	H *p. 216*	**39.**	E *p. 219*
32.	G *p. 215*	**36.**	J *p. 216*	**40.**	I *p. 223*
33.	C *p. 223*	**37.**	F *p. 216*		
34.	A *p. 225*	**38.**	B *p. 223*		

SHORT ANSWER

41. Positive end-expiratory pressure
42. Continuous positive airway pressure
43. Bilevel positive airway pressure
44. Chronic obstructive pulmonary disease
45. Acute respiratory distress syndrome
46. Positive-pressure ventilation
47. Vascular access device
48. Peripherally inserted central catheter
49. Do not attempt resuscitation orders
50. Congestive heart failure

Special Project

Answers will vary depending upon the agencies and hospices located in your area. You might want to discuss available services with the hospitals and health departments where you work. The information will not only familiarize you with home health care but also will provide a source of referral for patients who are unaware of these services.

Special Patients: Content Review

Content Self-Evaluation

CHAPTER 1: GYNECOLOGY

1.	B *p. 3*	**10.**	D *p. 6*	**19.**	B *p. 12*
2.	C *p. 5*	**11.**	C *p. 7*	**20.**	B *p. 12*
3.	B *p. 5*	**12.**	A *p. 8*	**21.**	B *p. 12*
4.	E *p. 5*	**13.**	E *p. 8*	**22.**	D *p. 13*
5.	A *p. 6*	**14.**	C *p. 8*	**23.**	A *p. 13*
6.	B *p. 6*	**15.**	D *p. 10*	**24.**	D *p. 13*
7.	A *p. 6*	**16.**	C *p. 10*	**25.**	E *p. 14*
8.	B *p. 6*	**17.**	B *p. 11*		
9.	C *p. 6*	**18.**	E *p. 11*		

CHAPTER 2: OBSTETRICS

26.	B *p. 19*	**33.**	E *p. 27*	**40.**	A *p. 38*
27.	C *p. 20*	**34.**	C *p. 27*	**41.**	C *p. 38*
28.	B *p. 22*	**35.**	C *p. 30*	**42.**	D *p. 39*
29.	D *p. 22*	**36.**	E *p. 32*	**43.**	A *p. 40*
30.	D *p. 22*	**37.**	A *p. 32*	**44.**	B *p. 41*
31.	C *p. 24*	**38.**	A *p. 33*	**45.**	A *p. 44*
32.	B *p. 24*	**39.**	B *p. 34*		

CHAPTER 3: NEONATOLOGY

46.	A *p. 49*	**50.**	D *p. 60*	**54.**	B *p. 66*
47.	C *p. 49*	**51.**	C *p. 63*	**55.**	D *p. 67*
48.	A *p. 53*	**52.**	E *p. 65*		
49.	E *p. 54*	**53.**	A *p. 66*		

CHAPTER 4: PEDIATRICS

56.	A *p. 72*	**69.**	C *p. 113*
57.	E *p. 73*	**70.**	B *p. 117*
58.	A *p. 74*	**71.**	E *p. 118*
59.	C *p. 74*	**72.**	A *p. 119*
60.	A *p. 84*	**73.**	A *p. 119*
61.	B *p. 88*	**74.**	C *p. 122*
62.	B *p. 88*	**75.**	B *p. 123*
63.	D *p. 93*	**76.**	D *p. 125*
64.	A *p. 99*	**77.**	E *p. 125*
65.	C *p. 98*	**78.**	B *p. 127*
66.	B *p. 112*	**79.**	E *p. 127*
67.	C *p. 102*	**80.**	B *p. 129*
68.	A *p. 106*		

CHAPTER 5: GERIATRIC EMERGENCIES

81.	A *p. 140*	**91.**	C *p. 162*
82.	B *p. 142*	**92.**	D *p. 163*
83.	B *p. 145*	**93.**	A *p. 166*
84.	E *p. 146*	**94.**	C *p. 163*
85.	D *p. 148*	**95.**	B *p. 164*
86.	C *p. 149*	**96.**	B *p. 165*
87.	E *p. 149*	**97.**	A *p. 167*
88.	A *p. 152*	**98.**	E *p. 168*
89.	B *p. 151*	**99.**	E *p. 170*
90.	E *p. 156*	**100.**	B *p. 179*

CHAPTER 6: ABUSE, NEGLECT, AND ASSAULT

101.	C *p. 184*	**106.**	B *p. 191*
102.	B *p. 186*	**107.**	A *p. 191*
103.	B *p. 187*	**108.**	B *p. 191*
104.	D *p. 189*	**109.**	A *p. 192*
105.	C *p. 190*	**110.**	D *p. 192*

CHAPTER 7: THE CHALLENGED PATIENT

111.	A *p. 198*	**116.**	B *p. 203*
112.	A *p. 199*	**117.**	A *p. 204*
113.	B *p. 199*	**118.**	A *p. 205*
114.	C *p. 200*	**119.**	D *p. 205*
115.	D *p. 202*	**120.**	A *p. 205*

CHAPTER 8: ACUTE INTERVENTIONS FOR THE CHRONIC CARE PATIENT

121.	E *p. 213*	**126.**	D *p. 227*
122.	C *p. 214*	**127.**	A *p. 230*
123.	B *p. 216*	**128.**	B *p. 230*
124.	D *p. 224*	**129.**	E *p. 230*
125.	A *p. 224*	**130.**	E *p. 230*

PATIENT SCENARIO FLASH CARDS

In order to help you learn the process of investigating the chief complaint and obtaining the past medical history, we have included a series of flash cards. Each one contains the dispatch and scene size-up information and then asks you to question either the patient's chief complaint or the past medical history.

Using the flash cards is a two-person exercise. Work with another member of your class, a paramedic or EMT from your service, or with someone else knowledgeable in emergency medical care. Cut the cards and shuffle them. Have your partner choose a card at random and read the dispatch and scene size-up information aloud to you. He should read the patient information to prepare to play the role of the patient. You should then try to determine the patient history by questioning him using the elements of the SAMPLE mnemonic. Your partner should then choose other cards and the two of you should repeat the exercise until you feel comfortable in gathering the patient history.

Then have your partner repeat the exercise, reading the dispatch and scene size-up information and role-playing the part of the patient with symptoms associated with the chief complaint. You should then question him about the chief complaint using the OPQRST-ASPN mnemonic. When you feel comfortable with the process of questioning for the chief complaint, repeat the exercise with your partner using information on both sides of the card. When you have gathered all the information you can, create a patient report like the one you would provide when arriving at the emergency department with your patient. Also attempt to determine the field diagnosis for the patient (listed at the bottom of the chief complaint card). Repeat the exercise until you are comfortable with the entire process.

PATIENT HISTORY

The patient history examines critical elements of the patient's past medical history, including the elements of the SAMPLE history mnemonic. (The S, for signs and symptoms, is investigated during the questioning about the chief complaint.)

A—allergies	Ask about any allergies or adverse reactions to drugs, foods, etc.
M—medications	Ask about any prescribed medications, then over-the-counter ones.
P—past medical history	Ask about recent surgeries, hospitalizations, and physician care.
L—last oral intake	Ask about the most recent meal and any fluids ingested.
E—events before the incident	Ask about activities and symptoms preceding the incident.

CHIEF COMPLAINT

During the investigation of the chief complaint, question the patient about the major symptoms of the problem to help form a field diagnosis. Investigate your patient's complaints by using the OPQRST-ASPN mnemonic.

O—onset	Ask about how the symptoms developed and what the patient was doing at the time.
P—palliation/provocation	Ask about what makes the symptoms better or worse.
Q—quality	Ask the patient to describe the nature of the pain or discomfort.
R—region/radiation	Ask where the symptom and related symptoms are found.
S—severity	Ask the patient to rate the pain on a scale from 1 to 10 (worst pain).
T—time	Ask about when the symptoms first appeared and how they progressed.
AS—associated symptoms	Ask about other or associated symptoms.
PN—pertinent negatives	Investigate likely and related signs and symptoms.

During this exercise, do not try to develop standard questions for each element of the investigation. Rather, let your patient's condition, the nature of the problem, and—later during your career—your experience guide your questioning to garner the pertinent medical information.

Scenario 1 Patient History

Dispatch Information: Responding to a residence for an unresponsive 2-week-old infant.

Scene Size-up: As your ambulance pulls up to a residential address, a teenage mother is crying while carrying her baby out to the ambulance; no hazards are apparent.

Medical History

A—she doesn't know of any

M—none

P—term pregnancy without complication

L—poor feeding for 2 days

E—elevated temperature today

Scenario 2 Patient History

Dispatch Information: Dispatched to a residence for complications of childbirth.

Scene Size-up: The father of a newly born infant leads you to a midwife. The midwife is attempting to resuscitate a blue-appearing newborn who is not breathing; no hazards are noted.

Medical History

A—unknown

M—none

P—normal pregnancy

L—none

E— at birth, neonate was apneic and unresponsive; mother's first-time labor and delivery

Scenario 3 Patient History

Dispatch Information: Dispatched to the parking lot of a local drug store where a car is standing by with an 18-month-old toddler having a seizure.

Scene Size-up: A young couple appears extremely upset as they direct your ambulance to their car; the car is running and traffic is busy in the parking lot.

Secure the Scene: Turn off the car's engine and have a crew member establish a safety perimeter using cones or scene tape.

Medical History

A—none

M—nonaspirin pain reliever

P—cold and upper respiratory congestion

L—last took medication about 2 hours ago

E—while driving, the father looked in the rearview mirror and saw the child's eyes roll back in her head and the mother observed total body shaking for approximately 30 seconds

Scenario 1 Chief Complaint "My Baby Is Sick."

O—Baby would not fully awaken from nap about 2 hours ago, has become less responsive

P—only a couple of ounces of formula today, no effect; Tylenol 2 hours ago, no improvement

Q—n/a

R—skin color is mottled, fontanelles are sunken

S—n/a

T—baby has been fussy for 2 days, developed fever today

AS—fewer diapers used in the last 24 hours

PN—no diarrhea or vomiting

(Field Diagnosis: Infection and Dehydration)

Scenario 2 Chief Complaint "The Baby Is Not Breathing."

O—at birth, neonate was apneic and unresponsive

P—n/a

Q—@1 minute—breathing slow and shallow, heart rate 100 (What is the APGAR score?)

@5 minutes—some spontaneous breathing, no other changes (What is the APGAR score?)

R—extremities blue, body pink, limp muscle tone

S—no response to stimuli or pain

T—normal and uneventful 14-hour delivery

AS—meconium staining noted

PN—term pregnancy w/no high-risk factors

(Field Diagnosis: Fetal Distress—Depressed Neonate)

Scenario 3 Chief Complaint "Seizures"

O—acute onset, first time, no warning (parents stopped car and loosened car seat straps)

P—n/a

Q—exaggerated body motion

R—whole body (arms, legs, torso, head)

S—n/a

T—recent cold and illness, 5 minutes after putting child in car seat

AS—now, skin very warm and moist, responds only to loud shouts

PN—no other seizure activity today or history of head trauma

(Field Diagnosis: Febrile Seizure)

Scenario 4 Patient History

Dispatch Information: Responding to a grocery market where a toddler has fallen from a shopping cart.

Scene Size-up: A small crowd is surrounding a woman holding a 2-year-old child. The child is crying and has an obvious goose egg on his forehead.

Medical History

A—penicillin

M—Dilantin

P—seizures

L—had lunch 30 minutes ago

E—child stood in shopping cart and fell out onto his head

Scenario 5 Patient History

Dispatch Information: Dispatched to a department store for an unconscious 68-year-old woman with a history of heart problems.

Scene Size-up: A crowd is gathered around an older woman who is lying on the floor, awake but disoriented.

Medical History

A—sulfa drugs and certain antibiotics

M—metaproterenol, isosorbide, and Miacalcin

P—hypertension, cardiac, and osteoporosis

L—nothing to eat today

E—shopping in the department store on a big sale day

Scenario 6 Patient History

Dispatch Information: Dispatched to a residence for a fall.

Scene Size-up: Apartment door is unlocked, and an older gentleman is calling out for help; no hazards noted.

Medical History

A—none

M—Lasix, nitro, potassium, Ventolin, and verapamil

P—cardiac, CHF, URI

L—had breakfast and took all medications right after

E—tripped and fell on scatter rug

Scenario 4 Chief Complaint "Fall with Head Impact"

O—sudden (mother had just turned away)

P—cries louder when bump is touched, mother can comfort child

Q—4-foot fall (cart to hard floor)

R—to anterior forehead

S—minor swelling, size of quarter

T—fall occurred 5 minutes ago

AS—none

PN—patient moves all extremities on mother's request

(Field Diagnosis: Head and Possible Neck Trauma)

Scenario 5 Chief Complaint "Dizziness, Collapse"

O—suddenly felt weak and dizzy while shopping, now somewhat confused

P—lying down, sitting increases dizziness and pulse rate

Q—dizzy and confused

R—n/a

S—oriented to persons, not to time or place

T—no previous episodes or warning for this one, can't remember why she is there

AS—pale, warm, moist skin; weak, irregular distal pulse

PN—no chest pain dyspnea, or signs of trauma

(Field Diagnosis: Undetermined, Rule Out Cardiac Syncope)

Scenario 6 Chief Complaint "Tripped, Can't Get Up."

O—pain in left hip after falling

P—pain is worse with movement and palpation

Q—constant severe pain

R—left hip and groin

S—pain is 9 on a scale of 1 to 10

T—while walking with a cane to the bathroom, tripped on the rug; pain came directly after fall

AS—left leg is shortened and medially rotated

PN—no loss of consciousness, weakness, or dizziness before or after the fall

(Field Diagnosis: Rule Out Fracture/Dislocation of Hip)

Scenario 7 Patient History

Dispatch Information: Domestic disturbance, police on scene.

Scene Size-up: Two police vehicles outside of single-family residence. A woman with cuts and bruises on her face and arms is being escorted to the ambulance; no other persons or hazards apparent.

Medical History

A—none

M—Zoloft, tramadol

P—depression and chronic back pain

L—last oral intake has been alcohol

E—patient and boyfriend got into a disagreement that turned physical

Scenario 8 Patient History

Dispatch Information: Dispatched to the nurse's office at a junior high school in reference to an assault.

Scene Size-up: Police are on the scene taking a report from teacher. The teacher was reportedly assaulted by a student; no hazards noted.

Medical History

A—environmental

M—none

P—diet-controlled diabetic

L—sandwich and cola for lunch 40 minutes ago

E—teacher attempted to break up a fistfight between two students

Scenario 9 Patient History

Dispatch Information: Dispatched to a motor vehicle collision; one patient with neck pain.

Scene Size-up: Upon arrival at a motor vehicle collision involving two cars, police direct you to a man complaining of chest pain and a woman who is "signing" to him. Both are standing in a driveway just off the road. Both are obese; no hazards noted.

Medical History

A—peanuts

M—none

P—deaf since birth

L—dinner an hour ago

E—patient's vehicle rear-ended another car at low speed, air bag deployed

Scenario 7 Chief Complaint "Domestic Disturbance"

O—police state neighbors report recent fighting and drinking (last hour), patient is evasive and inconsistent during interview

P—n/a

Q—significant developing hematoma to left cheek area (new)

R—numerous abrasions and minor lacerations over head, neck, and distal extremities (old)

S—minor trauma

T—old and new wounds

AS—none

PN—rest of assessment normal

(Field Diagnosis: Likely Long-Term Physical Abuse)

Scenario 8 Chief Complaint "Assault, Abdominal Pain"

O—abdominal pain has persisted after being kicked in the stomach by a student

P—pain has been getting progressively worse since incident

Q—sharp, intermittent, throbbing

R—pain is radiating around into the left flank area

S—pain is 8 on a scale of 1 to 10

T—incident occurred an hour ago

AS—nausea

PN—no vomiting

(Field Diagnosis: Internal Abdominal Hemorrhage)

Scenario 9 Chief Complaint "Chest Pain"

(Communication is slow due to writing down all Q&As).

O—immediate chest pain occurred after collision

P—pain is worse with inspiration and palpation

Q—pain is sharp and tearing in nature

R—diagonal across chest area covered by shoulder harness

S—5 on a scale of 1 to 10

T—distracted by glaring sunlight, her car struck the car stopped in front of her, deploying the driver's side air bag.

AS—difficulty breathing, anxiety, increased difficulties in communication and patient interview

PN—no back or neck pain (reliable reporter), no loss of consciousness

(Field Diagnosis: Musculoskeletal Pain—Rule Out Cardiac)

Scenario 10 Patient History

Dispatch Information: Dispatched to a nursing facility for a respiratory distress patient.

Scene Size-up: A 74-year-old female is unresponsive, lying in her bed. Gurgling respirations are audible from the doorway.

Medical History

A—penicillin

M—a three-page medication administration record is given to you by the staff

P—end-stage lung and brain cancer; CHF, hypertension, dementia

L—awake for small breakfast 4 hours ago

E—developed labored breathing and became progressively less responsive

Scenario 11 Patient History

Dispatch Information: Dispatched to a residence for a 4-year-old who has ingested an unknown product.

Scene Size-up: Neighbors lead you into the kitchen of a single-family dwelling. The father is washing the face of a 4-year-old girl in the kitchen sink. The child is crying weakly and has burns on her face, nose, and mouth. The mother shows you a milk container that contains an unknown gray liquid product.

Secure Scene: Have the mother take the product outside, but do not discard it. Open windows to air out the house and call for the fire department.

Medical History

A—none

M—none

P—asthma

L—last asthma attack was 3 months ago

E—the child was found screaming and crying in the garage

Scenario 12 Patient History

Dispatch Information: Dispatched to a remote farmhouse at the edge of the county line for a 75-year-old sick person.

Scene Size-up: After a 45-minute response, you arrive at a well-maintained farmhouse to find a 75-year-old woman with an altered mental status under the care of a registered nurse. The nurse reports that the patient has an elevated temperature and an increase in altered mental status today.

Medical History

A—codeine

M—levodopa, bromocriptine, and amantadine

P—Parkinson's disease

L—oral intake has been minimal for the past 24 hours

E—the central venous access port appears to be infected

Scenario 10 Chief Complaint "Unconscious"

O—unresponsive starting 30 minutes ago

P—n/a

Q—gurgling in upper airways, crackles in all lung fields

R—n/a

S—unresponsive to any stimuli

T—sudden onset of labored breathing 2 hours ago, progressive worsening

AS—pale skin, decreased SaO_2 and rapid, strong pulse

PN—no peripheral edema, oropharynx is clear

(Field Diagnosis: Exacerbation of COPD and CHF)

Scenario 11 Chief Complaint "Caustic Ingestion"

O—pain and crying immediately upon contact/attempted ingestion

P—face washed with water, reduced crying

Q—facial erythema, blistering, and edema

R—face, nose, lips, tongue, and mouth

S—obviously painful but with limited crying

T—child fine immediately before attempted ingestion

AS—parents upset by incident

PN—no wheezing or decreased breath sounds, no attempt at antidote administration, no nausea, posterior throat appears clear of burns

(Field Diagnosis: Accidental Caustic Ingestion with Facial Burns)

Scenario 12 Chief Complaint "Altered Mental Status"

O—decreasing LOC over last few hours

P—fever medications ineffective

Q—n/a

R—Port-A-Cath site inflamed

S—disoriented to time, place, and person

T—elevated temperature during the day, slow decrease in mental status over last few hours

AS—decreased urine output, mild tachycardia

PN—no respiratory disease, SaO_2 98 percent on room air

(Field Diagnosis: Systemic Infection)